THE COMPLETE LOW-CARB COOKBOOK

100+ Easy Recipes to Help You Eat Healthy and Stay on Track with Your Weight Loss Goals.

MILTON B. GRAHAM

Copyright © 2024 Milton B. Graham

CONTENTS

INTRODUCTION

The low-carbohydrate diet is one technique that has survived the test of time, achieving considerable popularity and praise for its probable health benefits. In a world where food trends are continuously evolving, this strategy has been demonstrated to be both effective and popular. There has never been a period when there has been a greater need for comprehensive resources that cater to certain dietary preferences than there is today. This is because individuals are increasingly wanting to take care of their well-being and make deliberate choices about their diet. Among the variety of culinary guides that are currently available, "The Complete LOW-CARB Cookbook" stands out as a brilliant example. This book claims to be more than merely a compilation of recipes; rather, it is a full guide to embracing and living on a route that requires eating fewer carbs.

This cookbook goes beyond the traditional bounds of a simple collection of recipes; rather, it is a compilation of culinary knowledge, nutritional insight, and practical guidance that is intended to empower persons who are beginning a lifestyle that is low in carbohydrates. This cookbook demystifies the low-carb strategy by paying rigorous attention to detail and dedicating it to both flavor and health. As a consequence, it is a technique that is accessible to both newcomers and seasoned lovers alike.

Within the pages of "The Complete LOW-CARB Cookbook," readers will find a range of scrumptious recipes that defy the popular misconception that a low-carb diet is connected with foods that are flavorless and dull. Every dish, from the most intriguing breakfast options to the most rewarding main meals, delectable desserts, and everything in between, is produced with the double purpose of delighting the taste buds and aligning with the principles of living a low-carbohydrate lifestyle. The cookbook assures that there is a broad range of possibilities to appeal to a variety of tastes and preferences, no matter if one follows a Ketogenic diet, an Atkins diet, or any other form of low-carb diet.

However, this cookbook is more than simply a compilation of recipes; it is a useful companion on the path toward a low-carb diet. It contains a wealth of information on the science underlying carbohydrate metabolism, the benefits of adopting a low-carb lifestyle, and practical recommendations for fitting this nutritional strategy into daily living in a manner that is both smooth and successful. It navigates the often confusing world of macronutrients with clarity and simplicity, allowing readers to make choices that are by their health and wellness goals by providing them with the required knowledge.

As we enter into the domain of "The Complete LOW-CARB Cookbook," we engage in a gastronomic adventure that surpasses the constraints of conventional diets. This isn't just about eliminating carbohydrates; it's about adopting a lifestyle that promotes prolonged health, vitality, and a renewed relationship with food. Whether you're a seasoned low-carb enthusiast or a newcomer curious about the prospective benefits, this cookbook is your trusted guide, guaranteeing that your route is not only nutritious but also delectable. Welcome to a world where low-carb living is not just a choice but a celebration of the rich tapestry of flavors that make a genuinely enjoyable and health-conscious culinary experience.

UNDERSTANDING LOW-CARB DIETS

Understanding low-carb diets is crucial for everyone attempting to adopt a healthy lifestyle or manage specific health conditions. Low-carb diets, as the name implies, prioritize decreasing the intake of carbohydrates while enhancing the consumption of proteins and fats. This dietary plan is based on the assumption that limiting carbs may lead to various health benefits, including weight loss, improved blood sugar control, and increased overall well-being.

At the core of low-carb diets is the idea of carbohydrate restriction. Carbohydrates are macronutrients present in foods including grains, fruits, vegetables, and legumes. When consumed, carbohydrates are broken down into glucose, which serves as the body's principal source of energy. However, excessive carb intake may lead to increases in blood sugar levels, which may contribute to weight gain, insulin resistance, and other metabolic diseases.

By reducing carb intake, low-carb diets strive to manage blood sugar levels and boost fat burning for energy instead of relying on glucose from carbohydrates. This metabolic state, known as ketosis, develops when the body begins to utilize stored fat for fuel, resulting in weight loss and healthier body composition.

There are different variations of low-carb diets, each with its particular ideas and recommendations. Some popular examples include the Ketogenic diet, which is extremely low in carbohydrates and high in fat, the Atkins diet, which gradually phases out carbs while raising protein and fat intake, and the paleo diet, which concentrates on whole, unprocessed meals while limiting grains and legumes.

Learning the basics of low-carb diets requires learning how to identify and choose meals that are low in carbohydrates while nonetheless offering critical nutrients. This typically entails prioritizing real foods including meat, fish, eggs, non-starchy vegetables, nuts, and seeds, while decreasing or eliminating processed meals, sugary snacks, and refined carbohydrates.

It's vital to note that while low-carb diets may be effective for weight loss and improving certain health markers, they may not be suitable for everyone. Individuals with special medical conditions or dietary restrictions should see a healthcare professional before making major changes to their diet.

In summary, comprehending low-carb diets includes recognizing the role of carbohydrates in the body, learning how carb restriction could influence metabolism and health, and adopting approaches for choosing nutrient-dense, low-carb meals. By adopting the ideas of low-carb eating, individuals may attain their health and wellness goals while enjoying a diverse and fun diet.

When entering into the domain of low-carb cooking, having the essential kitchen prerequisites may make all the difference in generating excellent and satisfying meals while being faithful to your nutritional aims. Here's a full list of kitchen essentials for low-carb cooking:

1. Quality Knives: A set of sharp knives is important for every kind of cooking, allowing you to effortlessly slice and dice vegetables, meats, and other components.

2. Cutting Boards: Invest in strong cutting boards to safeguard your countertops and ensure food safety while preparing low-carb products.

3. Vegetable Spiralizer: A spiralizer is a superb tool for transforming vegetables like zucchini, carrots, and squash into low-carb noodle substitutes, perfect for pasta replacements.

4. Food Processor or Blender: From blending creamy soups to churning up homemade sauces and dressings, a food processor or blender is important for producing delightful low-carb meals.

5. Cast Iron pan: A flexible and durable cast iron pan is great for sautéing vegetables, searing meats, and even preparing low-carb desserts like skillet cookies or brownies.

6. Non-Stick Pans: Non-stick pans are fantastic for cooking eggs, fish, and other delicate things without the need for extra oil or butter.

7. Baking Sheets and Pans: Stock your kitchen with baking sheets and pans for roasting vegetables, preparing low-carb bread, and cooking sheet pan meals.

8. Measuring Cups and Spoons: Accurate measurement is vital in low-carb cooking, so make sure you have a set of measuring cups and spoons for the proper portioning of ingredients.

9. Digital Kitchen Scale: A digital kitchen scale is vital for measuring ingredients by weight, especially when following low-carb recipes that need correct quantities.

10. Vegetable Steamer: Steaming veggies keep their nutrients and natural tastes, making a vegetable steamer a must-have for low-carb meal prep.

11. Grill or Grill Pan: Grilling is a healthy cooking method that delivers exceptional taste to meats, seafood, and vegetables without adding extra carbs.

12. Storage Containers: Keep your low-carb foods fresh and tidy using a variety of storage containers, including glass jars, Tupperware, and resealable bags.

13. Herbs and Spices: Build a well-stocked pantry with herbs, spices, and seasonings to offer depth and richness to your low-carb recipes without relying on high-carb sauces or condiments.

14. Healthy Fats: Stock up on healthy fats like olive oil, coconut oil, avocado oil, and grass-fed butter for cooking and flavoring low-carb foods.

15. Low-Carb Flours and Sweeteners: Explore alternative flours like almond flour, coconut flour, and flaxseed meal, as well as natural sweeteners like stevia, erythritol, and monk fruit for producing low-carb pleasures.

By equipping your kitchen with these essential tools and ingredients, you'll be well-prepared to embark on a delightful and fulfilling low-carb cooking journey. Whether you're whipping up speedy workday meals or indulging in tasty desserts, these kitchen staples will help you keep on track with your low-carb lifestyle aims.

BREAKFAST DELIGHTS

Avocado and Bacon Egg Cups

Prep time: 10 minutes | **Cook time**: 15-20 minutes | **Total time**: 25-30 minutes | **Serving size**: 6 egg cups

Ingredients:

- 3 ripe avocados
- 6 slices bacon, cooked and crumbled
- 6 eggs
- Salt and pepper to taste
- Optional toppings: chopped chives, shredded cheese, hot sauce

Directions:

1. Preheat oven to 400°F (200°C).

2. Cut the avocados in half and remove the pits.

3. Scoop out a small amount of avocado flesh from each half to create a nest for the egg. Don't go too deep, or the egg white will run out.

4. Place the avocado halves in a muffin tin.

5. Crack an egg into each avocado half.

6. Sprinkle with salt and pepper to taste.

7. Bake for 15-20 minutes, or until the egg whites are set and the yolks are cooked to your liking.

8. Top with crumbled bacon and your favorite toppings, if desired.

Nutritional information per serving: Calories: 220, Fat: 18g, Carbohydrates: 2g (net), Protein: 12g

Tips:

- If you like your eggs runny, bake for 12-15 minutes.
- For a creamier egg, whisk the eggs with a splash of milk or cream before adding them to the avocados.
- You can also add other low-carb ingredients to the egg cups, such as chopped vegetables, cheese, or sausage.

Spinach and Feta Omelette

Cooking time: 10 minutes | **Prep time**: 5 minutes | **Total time**: 15 minutes | **Serving size**: 1 omelette

Ingredients:

- 2 eggs
- 1/2 cup fresh spinach
- 1/4 cup crumbled feta cheese
- 1 tablespoon olive oil
- Salt and pepper to taste
- Optional: 1/4 teaspoon dried oregano or red pepper flakes

Directions:

1. Whisk together the eggs, salt, and pepper in a bowl.

2. Heat the olive oil in a non-stick skillet over medium heat.

3. Add the spinach and cook until wilted, about 1-2 minutes.

4. Pour in the egg mixture and tilt the pan to spread the eggs evenly.

5. Let the omelette cook for about 3 minutes, or until the bottom is set.

6. Sprinkle the feta cheese over one half of the omelette.

7. Using a spatula, fold the other half of the omelette over the filling.

8. Cook for another minute, or until the omelette is cooked through.

9. Slide the omelette onto a plate and serve immediately.

Nutritional information per serving: Calories: 250, Fat: 18g, Carbohydrates: 2g (net), Protein: 20g

Tips:

- For an extra burst of flavor, add a chopped shallot or clove of garlic to the pan with the spinach.
- If you don't have fresh spinach, you can use frozen spinach that has been thawed and squeezed dry.
- You can also add other low-carb vegetables to the omelette, such as mushrooms, bell peppers, or onions.
- Serve the omelette with a side of avocado slices or salsa for a complete meal.

Keto Pancakes

Cooking Time: 10-12 minutes | **Prep Time**: 5 minutes | **Total Time**: 15-17 minutes | **Serving Size**: 6

Ingredients:

- 1/2 cup almond flour
- 1/4 cup coconut flour
- 1 teaspoon baking powder
- 1/4 teaspoon salt
- 2 eggs
- 1/4 cup unsweetened almond milk
- 1 tablespoon melted coconut oil
- 1/2 teaspoon vanilla extract
- Optional: Monk fruit sweetener or sugar substitute, to taste

Directions:

1. Whisk dry ingredients: In a medium bowl, whisk together the almond flour, coconut flour, baking powder, and salt.
2. Combine wet ingredients: In a separate bowl, whisk together the eggs, almond milk, coconut oil, and vanilla extract.
3. Combine wet and dry ingredients: Pour the wet ingredients into the dry ingredients and gently fold until just combined. Be careful not to over mix, as this can make the pancakes tough.
4. Heat pan: Heat a non-stick skillet over medium heat.
5. Cook pancakes: Pour 1/4 cup of batter per pancake onto the hot skillet. Cook for 2-3 minutes per side, or until golden brown.
6. Serve: Serve immediately with your favorite low-carb toppings, such as sugar-free syrup, almond butter, fresh berries, or whipped cream.

Nutritional Information per pancake: Calories: 130, Fat: 9g, Carbohydrates: 5g (net 2g), Protein: 7g

Tips:

- For extra fluffy pancakes, let the batter rest for 5 minutes before cooking.
- If the batter is too thick, add a little more almond milk. If it's too thin, add a tablespoon or two of almond flour.
- You can also add in your favorite low-carb mix-ins, such as chopped nuts, chia seeds, or shredded coconut.
- Store leftover pancakes in an airtight container in the refrigerator for up to 3 days.

Chia Seed Pudding

Cooking Time: 0 minutes | **Prep Time**: 5 minutes | **Total Time**: 5 minutes | **Serving size**: 1

Ingredients:

- 1/4 cup chia seeds
- 1 cup unsweetened almond milk (or other low-carb milk like coconut milk)
- 1/2 teaspoon vanilla extract (optional)
- 1/4 teaspoon ground cinnamon (optional)
- Sweetener of choice (optional, such as stevia, monk fruit sweetener, or erythritol)
- Toppings of your choice (optional, such as berries, nuts, seeds, shredded coconut, or a drizzle of low-carb chocolate sauce)

Directions:

1. In a small bowl or Mason jar, combine the chia seeds, almond milk, vanilla extract (if using), and cinnamon (if using). Stir well to combine.

2. If using a sweetener, add it to the mixture and stir again.

3. Cover the bowl or jar and place it in the refrigerator. Let it sit for at least 2 hours, or preferably overnight, to allow the chia seeds to absorb the liquid and thicken up.

4. When ready to serve, stir the pudding again and top with your desired toppings. Enjoy!

Nutritional Information per serving: Calories: 280, Carbohydrates: 6g (3g net), Fiber: 10g, Protein: 8g, Fat: 18g

Tips:

- You can adjust the thickness of the pudding to your liking by adding more or less milk.
- For a richer flavor, use full-fat coconut milk instead of almond milk.
- Get creative with your toppings! Berries, nuts, seeds, and shredded coconut are all great options.
- If you like your pudding warm, you can heat it up gently in the microwave before serving.
- This pudding can be stored in the refrigerator for up to 3 days.

Baked Egg Muffins

Prep Time: 10 minutes | **Cooking Time**: 20-25 minutes | **Total Time**: 30-35 minutes | **Serving Size**: 12

Ingredients:

- 8 large eggs
- 1/4 cup unsweetened almond milk (or regular milk if not low-carb)
- 1/2 teaspoon dried oregano
- 1/4 teaspoon garlic powder
- Salt and pepper to taste

Optional mix-ins (choose 2-3):
- 1/2 cup chopped ham or diced cooked sausage
- 1/2 cup chopped spinach or bell peppers
- 1/4 cup crumbled feta cheese
- 1/4 cup shredded cheddar cheese
- 1/4 cup chopped sun-dried tomatoes
- 1/4 cup chopped olives

Directions:

1. Preheat oven to 375°F (190°C). Grease a 12-cup muffin tin with cooking spray or line with silicone liners.

2. In a large bowl, whisk together eggs, almond milk, oregano, garlic powder, salt, and pepper.

3. Divide the egg mixture evenly among the muffin cups. Add your chosen mix-ins to each cup as desired.

4. Bake for 20-25 minutes, or until the eggs are set and golden brown around the edges.

5. Let cool in the pan for 5-10 minutes before serving. Muffins can be stored in an airtight container in the refrigerator for up to 3 days or frozen for up to 3 months.

Nutritional Information per Muffin: Calories: 130, Fat: 8 grams, Protein: 8 grams, Net Carbs: 1.5 grams

Tips:

- For extra flavor, use pre-cooked vegetables like sautéed onions or peppers.
- If you don't have almond milk, you can use water or another low-carb milk substitute.
- Get creative with your mix-ins! Any combination of vegetables, meats, and cheeses will work.
- These muffins can be easily reheated in the microwave for a quick and easy breakfast or snack.

Greek Yogurt Parfait

Cooking Time: 0 minutes | **Prep Time**: 5 minutes | **Total Time**: 5 minutes | **Serving size**: 1

Ingredients:

- 1 cup plain Greek yogurt (full-fat or 2% fat)
- 1/2 cup berries (strawberries, blueberries, raspberries, or blackberries)
- 1/4 cup chopped nuts or seeds (almonds, walnuts, pecans, pumpkin seeds, sunflower seeds)
- 1 tablespoon unsweetened shredded coconut
- 1/4 teaspoon cinnamon (optional)
- Stevia or monk fruit sweetener to taste (optional)

Directions:

1. In a bowl or parfait glass, layer half of the yogurt.

2. Top with half of the berries.

3. Sprinkle with half of the nuts or seeds and half of the shredded coconut.

4. Repeat layers with remaining yogurt, berries, nuts or seeds, and coconut.

5. Drizzle with stevia or monk fruit sweetener to taste (optional).

6. Sprinkle with cinnamon if desired.

Nutritional Information per serving: Calories: 300, Fat: 15g, Carbohydrates: 5g (net carbs), Fiber: 3g, Protein: 25g

Tips:

- For a creamier parfait, stir in a tablespoon of almond milk or heavy cream to the yogurt.
- If you don't have fresh berries, you can use frozen berries that have been thawed.
- You can also add other low-carb fruits to the parfait, such as melon or grapefruit.
- For a thicker parfait, let the chia seeds sit in the yogurt for 5 minutes before layering.
- Store any leftover parfait in the refrigerator for up to 2 days.

Berry Green Dream Smoothie

Cooking time: 0 minutes | **Prep time**: 5 minutes | **Total time**: 5 minutes | **Serving size**: 1 smoothie

Ingredients:

- 1/2 cup frozen berries (strawberries, blueberries, raspberries, or a mix)
- 1 cup unsweetened almond milk
- 1/2 cup spinach
- 1/4 avocado, peeled and chopped
- 1 tablespoon chia seeds
- 1 scoop vanilla protein powder (optional)
- 1/2 teaspoon vanilla extract
- 1/4 cup ice cubes (optional)

Directions:

1. Add all ingredients to a blender.

2. Blend until smooth and creamy.

3. Add more almond milk or ice cubes if desired for a thinner consistency.

4. Pour into a glass and enjoy!

Nutritional information per serving: Calories: 240, Carbohydrates: 6 grams (net carbs), Fiber: 4 grams, Protein: 15 grams, Fat: 14 grams

Tips:

- Use frozen berries for a thicker and colder smoothie.
- If you don't have protein powder, you can add a tablespoon of almond butter or peanut butter for extra protein and healthy fats.
- You can also add other low-carb vegetables to this smoothie, such as kale, cucumber, or celery.
- If you are on a strict keto diet, you may want to omit the banana and use all frozen berries.

Smoked Salmon Roll-Ups

Cooking Time: 5 minutes | **Prep Time**: 10 minutes | **Total Time**: 15 minutes | **Serving Size**: 10 roll-ups

Ingredients:

- 4 oz thinly sliced smoked salmon
- 4 oz softened cream cheese, whipped or Neufchatel cheese
- 2 Tbsp chopped fresh chives
- 1/2 Tbsp lemon juice
- 1/4 tsp black pepper
- 10 large lettuce leaves (romaine or butter lettuce work well)

Optional Add-Ins:

- Diced avocado
- Thinly sliced cucumber
- Chopped dill
- Everything bagel seasoning

Directions:

1. Soften the cream cheese: If your cream cheese is not already softened, microwave it in 15-second intervals until spreadable.
2. Combine the filling: In a small bowl, mix together the cream cheese, chives, lemon juice, and black pepper until smooth.
3. Assemble the roll-ups: Lay out a lettuce leaf on a plate. Spread about 1 tablespoon of the cream cheese mixture onto the lettuce leaf. Place a slice of smoked salmon on top of the cream cheese.
4. Add extras (optional): If using, sprinkle on your desired add-ins like avocado, cucumber, dill, or everything bagel seasoning.
5. Roll it up: Tightly roll up the lettuce leaf and salmon together, starting from the short end. Repeat with remaining ingredients to make 10 roll-ups.
6. Chill (optional): For a firmer texture, refrigerate the roll-ups for 30 minutes before serving.

Nutritional Information per Serving: Calories: 120, Fat: 5g, Carbohydrates: 1g (net), Protein: 14g

Tips:

- Use high-quality smoked salmon for the best flavor.
- If you don't have lettuce leaves, you can use nori seaweed wraps or thinly sliced cucumber as alternatives.
- Make the roll-ups ahead of time and store them in the refrigerator for up to 2 days.
- Get creative with the add-ins! Other options include diced red onion, capers, or crumbled feta cheese.

Cauliflower Hash Browns

Prep Time: 10 minutes | **Cooking Time**: 15 minutes | **Total Time**: 25 minutes | **Servings**: 4-6 patties

Ingredients:

- 1 head cauliflower, grated (about 4 cups)
- 1 large egg
- 1/4 cup almond flour
- 1/4 cup grated Parmesan cheese
- 1/4 teaspoon onion powder
- 1/4 teaspoon garlic powder
- Salt and pepper to taste
- Coconut oil or avocado oil for frying

Directions:

1. Prep the cauliflower: Grate the cauliflower using a box grater or food processor. Pulse until it resembles rice-sized pieces.
2. Squeeze out moisture: Transfer the grated cauliflower to a clean kitchen towel and wring out as much liquid as possible. This is crucial for achieving crispy hash browns.
3. Mix the dry ingredients: In a large bowl, combine the almond flour, Parmesan cheese, onion powder, garlic powder, salt, and pepper.
4. Incorporate the wet ingredients: Add the grated cauliflower and egg to the bowl and mix well until everything is evenly combined.
5. Form the patties: Scoop about 1/4 cup of the mixture and gently press it into a patty shape. Repeat with the remaining mixture, making sure not to overcrowd the pan.
6. Heat the oil: Heat a skillet over medium heat and add just enough oil to coat the bottom.
7. Cook the hash browns: Carefully add the patties to the pan and cook for 3-4 minutes per side, or until golden brown and crispy.
8. Drain and serve: Drain the hash browns on a paper towel to remove excess oil. Serve immediately with your favorite low-carb breakfast toppings, such as avocado slices, fried eggs, or a dollop of Greek yogurt.

Nutritional Information per serving: Calories: 130, Fat: 8g, Carbohydrates: 5g (net carbs 2g), Fiber: 3g, Protein: 6g

Tips:

- For extra flavor, add chopped fresh herbs like chives or parsley to the batter.
- If the mixture seems too wet, add a little more almond flour or shredded cheese.
- You can bake the hash browns instead of frying them. Preheat your oven to 400°F (200°C) and bake for 15-20 minutes, flipping halfway through.
- These hash browns are delicious leftovers! Store them in an airtight container in the refrigerator for up to 3 days.

Keto Breakfast Burrito

Prep Time: 10 minutes | **Cook Time**: 15 minutes | **Total Time**: 25 minutes | **Servings**: 2 burritos

Ingredients:

- 2 low-carb tortillas (such as Mission Carb Balance or Ole! Xtreme Wellness)
- 4 eggs
- 1/4 cup chopped onion
- 1/4 cup chopped bell pepper
- 3 slices bacon, cooked and crumbled
- 1/2 cup shredded cheddar cheese
- 1/4 avocado, sliced
- Salt and pepper to taste

Optional toppings:

- Salsa
- Hot sauce
- Sour cream

Directions:

1. Heat a skillet over medium heat. Add the onion and bell pepper and cook until softened, about 5 minutes.

2. In a separate bowl, whisk together the eggs with salt and pepper. Pour the egg mixture into the skillet with the vegetables and cook until scrambled, about 5 minutes.

3. Warm the tortillas according to package instructions. To assemble the burritos, spread a layer of scrambled eggs down the center of each tortilla. Top with bacon, cheese, avocado, and any desired toppings. Roll up the burritos and enjoy!

Nutritional Information per burrito: Calories: 450, Fat: 35g, Protein: 30g, Net Carbs: 5g

Tips

- For a vegetarian option, omit the bacon and use crumbled tofu or tempeh instead.
- You can also make these burritos ahead of time and store them in the refrigerator for up to 3 days.
- To freeze the burritos, wrap them tightly in plastic wrap and then aluminum foil. Freeze for up to 3 months. Thaw overnight in the refrigerator before reheating.

Coconut Flour Waffles

Prep Time: 5 minutes | **Cooking Time**: 7-10 minutes | **Total Time**: 12-15 minutes | **Servings**: 2 waffles

Ingredients:

- 1/4 cup coconut flour, sifted
- 2 tablespoons almond flour
- 1 teaspoon baking powder
- 1/4 teaspoon sea salt
- 2 large eggs
- 1/4 cup unsweetened almond milk
- 1 tablespoon melted coconut oil
- 1/2 teaspoon vanilla extract
- Optional: 1/4 teaspoon cinnamon or other spices

Directions:

1. In a medium bowl, whisk together the coconut flour, almond flour, baking powder, and salt.

2. In a separate bowl, whisk together the eggs, almond milk, coconut oil, vanilla extract, and any optional spices.

3. Pour the wet ingredients into the dry ingredients and whisk until just combined. Don't over mix! The batter will be thick.

4. Preheat your waffle iron to medium heat. Grease the waffle iron if needed.

5. Pour about 1/2 cup of batter into each waffle iron section. Close the lid and cook for 7-10 minutes, or until golden brown and crispy.

6. Serve immediately with your favorite low-carb toppings.

Nutritional Information per waffle: Calories: 240, Fat: 20g, Carbohydrates: 5g (net carbs 2g), Protein: 10g, Fiber: 3g

Tips:

- To make sure your waffles don't stick, preheat your waffle iron well and grease it lightly with coconut oil or avocado oil.
- Don't over mix the batter! Over mixing will make the waffles tough.
- If the batter is too thick, add a tablespoon or two of almond milk until it reaches a pourable consistency.
- Get creative with your toppings! These waffles are delicious with fresh berries, whipped cream, nuts, seeds, or a drizzle of sugar-free syrup.

Caprese Salad

Prep Time: 5 minutes | **Cooking Time**: 0 minutes | **Total Time**: 5 minutes | **Serving Size**: 1

Ingredients:

- 2 medium tomatoes, sliced
- 4 ounces fresh mozzarella cheese, sliced or cubed
- 1/4 cup fresh basil leaves, chopped
- 1 tablespoon extra-virgin olive oil
- 1/2 teaspoon balsamic vinegar (optional)
- Salt and pepper to taste

Directions:

1. Slice the tomatoes and mozzarella cheese. Aim for even thickness for both.

2. Arrange the tomato slices on a plate. Top with the mozzarella cheese slices.

3. Scatter the chopped basil leaves over the salad. Drizzle with olive oil and balsamic vinegar (if using).

4. Season with salt and pepper to taste. Serve immediately and enjoy!

Nutritional Information per serving: Calories: 240, Fat: 18g, Carbohydrates: 5g (net 3g), Protein: 15g, Fiber: 2g

Tips:

- For a heartier breakfast, add a protein element like sliced smoked salmon, grilled chicken, or hard-boiled eggs.
- If you're short on time, use cherry tomatoes that don't need slicing.
- Get creative with the presentation! Arrange the ingredients in a beautiful pattern or serve the salad in individual mason jars.
- Store any leftover salad in an airtight container in the refrigerator for up to 24 hours.

Keto Breakfast Casserole

Cooking time: 35 minutes | **Prep time**: 10 minutes | **Total time**: 45 minutes | **Servings**: 8-10

Ingredients:

- 1 tablespoon olive oil
- 1 pound ground sausage (pork, turkey, or chicken)
- 1/2 bell pepper, chopped
- 1/2 onion, chopped
- 1 clove garlic, minced
- 8 large eggs
- 1 cup heavy cream
- 1/2 teaspoon salt
- 1/4 teaspoon black pepper
- 1 cup shredded cheddar cheese
- 1/2 cup chopped spinach (optional)
- 1/4 cup chopped sun-dried tomatoes (optional)

Directions:

1. Preheat oven to 375°F (190°C). Grease an 8x8 inch baking dish.
2. Heat olive oil in a large skillet over medium heat. Add ground sausage and cook until browned, breaking it up with a spoon. Drain any excess fat.
3. Add bell pepper, onion, and garlic to the skillet and cook until softened, about 5 minutes.
4. In a large bowl, whisk together eggs, heavy cream, salt, and pepper. Stir in cooked sausage and vegetables.
5. If using, stir in spinach and sun-dried tomatoes.
6. Pour the egg mixture into the prepared baking dish. Sprinkle with cheddar cheese.
7. Bake for 35-40 minutes, or until eggs are set and cheese is melted.
8. Let cool slightly before serving.

Nutritional information per serving: Calories: 320, Fat: 24g, Protein: 25g, Net carbs: 4g

Tips:

- Feel free to customize this recipe with your favorite low-carb ingredients. Other good options include broccoli, mushrooms, zucchini, and ham.
- You can also make this casserole ahead of time. Simply assemble it the night before and bake in the morning.
- For a heartier casserole, add cooked bacon or chorizo.
- Serve this casserole with a side of avocado slices or low-carb salsa.

Egg and Bacon Roll-Ups

Cooking Time: 15 minutes | **Prep Time**: 10 minutes | **Total Time**: 25 minutes | **Serving Size**: 4 roll-ups

Ingredients:

- 4 slices bacon
- 2 large eggs
- 1/4 cup shredded cheddar cheese
- 1 tablespoon chopped chives (optional)
- Salt and pepper to taste

Directions:

1. Cook the bacon: Fry the bacon slices in a skillet over medium heat until crispy. Drain on paper towels and set aside.

2. Scramble the eggs: In the same skillet used for the bacon, whisk together the eggs. Season with salt and pepper. Scramble the eggs over medium heat until just cooked through.

3. Assemble the roll-ups: Lay out a bacon slice on a plate. Sprinkle with some cheddar cheese and chives (if using). Top with a portion of scrambled eggs. Carefully roll up the bacon, securing the filling inside. Repeat with the remaining ingredients.

4. Optional: To add a bit of crispness, bake the roll-ups on a baking sheet at 375°F for 5-7 minutes.

Nutritional Information per Roll-Up: Calories: 180, Fat: 13g, Carbohydrates: 1g, Fiber: 0g, Protein: 15g

Tips:

- For variety, you can add other low-carb ingredients to the filling, such as chopped spinach, mushrooms, or bell peppers.
- If you're short on time, you can use pre-cooked bacon or sausage.
- These roll-ups can be made ahead of time and stored in the refrigerator for up to 3 days. Reheat them in the microwave or oven before serving.

Zucchini Noodles with Pesto

Cooking Time: 5 minutes | **Prep Time**: 10 minutes | **Total Time**: 15 minutes | **Serving Size**: 1 person

Ingredients:

- 1 medium zucchini, spiralized or julienned
- 1/4 cup basil pesto (low-carb, store-bought or homemade)
- 1 tablespoon olive oil
- 1/4 cup cherry tomatoes, halved (optional)
- 1/4 cup crumbled feta cheese (optional)
- Freshly ground black pepper, to taste
- Pinch of red pepper flakes (optional)

Directions:

1. Prepare the zucchini: Wash and dry the zucchini. Using a spiralizer or julienne peeler, create long, thin noodles. Alternatively, you can thinly slice the zucchini into ribbons.

2. Cook the zucchini (optional): If you prefer your noodles with a slightly softened texture, heat the olive oil in a large skillet over medium heat. Add the zucchini noodles and cook for 2-3 minutes, stirring occasionally, until just tender-crisp. Do not overcook, or they will become mushy.

3. Mix the pesto: In a large bowl, toss the cooked or raw zucchini noodles with the pesto. If using raw noodles, the heat from the pesto will slightly soften them.

4. Assemble and serve: Divide the zucchini noodles with pesto between two plates. Top with cherry tomatoes, feta cheese, black pepper, and red pepper flakes (if using). Enjoy immediately!

Nutritional Information per serving: Calories: 240, Carbohydrates: 8g (net), Fiber: 3g, Fat: 14g, Protein: 8g

Tips:

- For a creamier sauce, add a splash of unsweetened almond milk or water to the pesto before tossing with the noodles.
- Substitute the basil pesto with a low-carb alternative like kale pesto or walnut pesto.
- Add sliced avocado or chopped spinach for extra nutrients and flavor.
- Leftovers can be stored in an airtight container in the refrigerator for up to 2 days. However, the noodles may become a bit watery, so it's best to enjoy them fresh.

Keto Avocado Smoothie

Prep Time: 5 minutes | **Cooking Time**: 0 minutes | **Total Time**: 5 minutes | **Servings**: 1

Ingredients:

- 1/2 ripe avocado, pitted and chopped
- 1 cup unsweetened almond milk
- 1/2 cup spinach
- 1 scoop vanilla or chocolate keto protein powder (optional)
- 1 tablespoon chia seeds
- 1/2 teaspoon vanilla extract
- 1/4 cup ice cubes (optional, depending on desired thickness)

Directions:

1. Add all ingredients to a high-powered blender.

2. Blend until smooth and creamy, about 30 seconds.

3. Pour into a glass and enjoy immediately!

Nutritional Information per Serving: Calories: 350, Fat: 30 g, Protein: 6 g, Carbs: 5 g (Net Carbs: 2 g), Fiber: 3 g, Sugar: 1 g

Tips:

- For an extra creamy texture, use frozen avocado chunks.
- You can also use other low-carb fruits or vegetables, such as berries, kale, or zucchini.
- Add a teaspoon of cocoa powder or matcha powder for a flavor boost.
- Top with your favorite keto-friendly toppings, such as whipped cream, chopped nuts, or seeds.

Egg and Sausage Breakfast Bites

Cooking Time: 20-25 minutes | **Prep Time**: 10 minutes | **Total Time**: 30 minutes | **Serving Size**: 12 bites

Ingredients:

- 12 oz ground breakfast sausage
- 6 eggs
- 1/2 cup shredded cheddar cheese
- 1/4 cup chopped bell pepper (optional)
- 1/4 cup chopped onion (optional)
- 1/4 teaspoon salt
- 1/4 teaspoon black pepper
- 1/8 teaspoon garlic powder
- Non-stick cooking spray

Directions:

1. Preheat oven to 350°F (175°C). Grease a muffin tin with non-stick cooking spray.

2. In a large skillet, brown the sausage over medium heat, breaking it up with a spoon. Drain any excess fat.

3. In a medium bowl, whisk together the eggs, cheese, bell pepper, onion, salt, pepper, and garlic powder.

4. Divide the sausage evenly among the muffin cups. Pour the egg mixture over the sausage, filling each cup almost to the top.

5. Bake for 20-25 minutes, or until the eggs are set and the cheese is melted.

6. Let cool slightly before serving.

Nutritional Information per bite: Calories: 130, Fat: 8g, Carbs: 1g, Protein: 12g

Tips:

- For a spicier bite, add a pinch of cayenne pepper to the egg mixture.
- You can also use other types of cheese, such as mozzarella or Monterey Jack.
- If you don't have a muffin tin, you can use mini ramekins or a greased baking dish.
- These bites can be stored in an airtight container in the refrigerator for up to 3 days.

Keto Bagel with Cream Cheese

Prep Time: 10 minutes | **Cooking Time**: 15 minutes | **Total Time**: 25 minutes | **Servings**: 2 bagels

Ingredients:

- 1 1/2 cups almond flour
- 1 tablespoon baking powder
- 3 cups shredded mozzarella cheese
- 2 ounces cream cheese, softened
- 3 large eggs, divided
- 1 tablespoon sesame seeds (optional)
- Everything Bagel Seasoning (optional)

Directions:

1. Preheat oven to 350°F (175°C). Line a baking sheet with parchment paper.

2. In a small bowl, whisk together almond flour and baking powder.

3. In a microwave-safe bowl, melt mozzarella cheese and cream cheese together in 30-second intervals, stirring until smooth.

4. Transfer the cheese mixture to a food processor. Add 2 eggs and the dry ingredients. Pulse until a dough forms.

5. Lightly flour a surface with almond flour. Divide the dough into two equal portions. Roll each portion into a long rope, then connect the ends to form a bagel shape.

6. Place the bagels on the prepared baking sheet. Brush with the remaining egg and sprinkle with sesame seeds and everything Bagel Seasoning, if desired.

7. Bake for 15-20 minutes, or until golden brown. Let cool slightly before slicing and spreading with cream cheese.

Nutritional Information per bagel: Calories: 240, Fat: 18g, Protein: 15g, Carbohydrates: 4g (net 2g)\, Fiber: 2g

Tips:

- For a softer bagel, bake for 15 minutes. For a chewier bagel, bake for 20 minutes.
- You can store leftover bagels in an airtight container in the refrigerator for up to 3 days. Reheat in the microwave or toaster before serving.
- Get creative with your toppings! Try avocado, smoked salmon, or your favorite keto-friendly spreads.

Broccoli and Cheese Frittata

Cooking time: 15-20 minutes | **Prep time**: 10 minutes | **Total time**: 25-30 minutes | **Servings**: 4-6 wedges

Ingredients:

- 8 large eggs
- 1/2 cup unsweetened almond milk (or heavy cream for higher fat content)
- 1/2 teaspoon dried oregano
- Salt and freshly ground black pepper to taste
- 1 tablespoon olive oil
- 1/2 yellow onion, diced
- 1 clove garlic, minced
- 1 head broccoli, cut into florets
- 1/2 cup shredded cheddar cheese

Directions:

1. Preheat oven to 350°F (175°C).

2. In a large bowl, whisk together eggs, almond milk, oregano, salt, and pepper.

3. Heat olive oil in a large oven-safe skillet over medium heat. Add onion and cook until softened, about 5 minutes.

4. Add garlic and cook for another minute until fragrant.

5. Add broccoli and cook for 2-3 minutes until slightly tender-crisp.

6. Pour the egg mixture into the skillet and top with cheese.

7. Transfer skillet to the oven and bake for 15-20 minutes, or until eggs are set and cheese is melted and bubbly.

8. Let cool slightly before cutting into wedges and serving.

Nutritional information per serving: Calories: 250, Fat: 18g, Carbohydrates: 5g (2g net carbs), Protein: 20g

Tips:
- For a richer flavor, use full-fat cheese and heavy cream.
- Add other low-carb vegetables like spinach, mushrooms, or bell peppers.
- Leftovers can be stored in an airtight container in the refrigerator for up to 3 days. Reheat gently in a skillet or microwave.
- This frittata is also delicious cold for a grab-and-go breakfast.

Low-Carb Breakfast Pizza

Prep Time: 10 minutes | **Cooking Time**: 20 minutes | **Total Time**: 30 minutes | **Serving Size**: 1 pizza

Ingredients:

Crust:
- 8 large eggs
- 1/4 cup heavy cream
- 1/2 teaspoon salt
- 1/4 teaspoon black pepper

Toppings:
- 4 ounces cooked breakfast sausage, crumbled
- 1/2 cup bell peppers, thinly sliced
- 1/2 cup cherry tomatoes, sliced
- 1 cup shredded cheddar cheese
- 1/4 cup chopped fresh spinach (optional)
- 1 tablespoon chopped fresh chives (optional)

Directions:

1. Preheat oven to 400°F (200°C). Line a baking sheet with parchment paper.

2. Prepare the crust: In a large bowl, whisk together eggs, cream, salt, and pepper until well combined. Pour the mixture onto the prepared baking sheet and spread evenly into a 12-inch circle.

3. Bake for 10-12 minutes, or until the crust is golden brown and set.

4. Remove from the oven and top with breakfast sausage, bell peppers, and tomatoes.

5. Return to the oven and bake for another 5-7 minutes, or until the cheese is melted and bubbly.

6. Garnish with spinach and chives (optional) and serve immediately.

Nutritional Information per slice: Calories: 350, Fat: 25g, Net Carbs: 4g, Protein: 25g

Tips:

- For a thicker crust, pre-bake the egg mixture for 5 minutes before adding toppings.
- Use different vegetables like onions, mushrooms, or broccoli for variation.
- Add protein variations like sliced turkey, ham, or cooked shrimp.
- Spice things up with a sprinkle of your favorite low-carb spices like red pepper flakes or Italian seasoning.
- Leftovers can be stored in an airtight container in the refrigerator for up to 3 days. Reheat in the oven or microwave until warmed through.

LUNCH

Grilled Chicken Salad

Prep time: 10 minutes | **Cooking time**: 15 minutes | **Total time**: 25 minutes | **Serving size**: 1

Ingredients:

- 1 boneless, skinless chicken breast
- 1 tablespoon olive oil
- 1/2 teaspoon salt
- 1/4 teaspoon black pepper
- 2 cups mixed greens
- 1/2 cup cherry tomatoes
- 1/4 cup crumbled feta cheese
- 2 tablespoons avocado dressing

Directions:

1. Preheat a grill to medium-high heat.

2. Drizzle the chicken breast with olive oil and season with salt and pepper.

3. Grill the chicken breast for 5-7 minutes per side, or until cooked through.

4. While the chicken is grilling, prepare the salad by adding the mixed greens, cherry tomatoes, and feta cheese to a bowl.

5. Once the chicken is cooked, slice it into strips and add it to the salad.

6. Drizzle the salad with avocado dressing and toss to combine.

7. Serve immediately.

Nutritional information: Calories: 350, Fat: 20g, Carbohydrates: 5g, Fiber: 2g, Protein: 30g

Tips:
- You can use any type of chicken you like, such as thighs or tenders.
- If you don't have a grill, you can cook the chicken in a skillet over medium heat.
- For a more flavorful salad, you can marinate the chicken in your favorite marinade for 30 minutes before grilling.
- You can also add other vegetables to the salad, such as cucumbers, onions, or avocado.
- If you don't have avocado dressing, you can use another low-carb dressing, such as vinaigrette or ranch.

Zucchini Noodles with Pesto

Cooking time: 5 minutes | **Prep time**: 15 minutes | **Total time**: 20 minutes | **Serving size**: 2

Ingredients:

- 2 medium zucchini
- 1/2 cup fresh basil leaves
- 1/4 cup pine nuts
- 1/4 cup grated Parmesan cheese
- 2 tablespoons olive oil
- 1/2 lemon, juiced
- 1 clove garlic, minced
- Salt and pepper to taste

Optional additions:

- Grilled chicken or shrimp
- Cherry tomatoes
- Sliced avocado
- Chopped bell peppers

Directions:

1. Spiralize the zucchini. Using a spiralizer, julienne peeler, or mandoline, create long, thin noodles from the zucchini. If you don't have a spiralizer, you can cut the zucchini into thin strips with a knife.
2. Make the pesto. In a food processor, combine the basil, pine nuts, Parmesan cheese, olive oil, lemon juice, garlic, salt, and pepper. Blend until smooth.
3. Cook the zucchini noodles (optional). If you prefer your noodles warmer, heat a tablespoon of olive oil in a large skillet over medium heat. Add the zucchini noodles and cook for 2-3 minutes, until slightly softened.
4. Assemble the dish. In a large bowl, toss the zucchini noodles with the pesto. Add any desired toppings, such as grilled chicken, shrimp, tomatoes, avocado, or bell peppers.
5. Serve immediately. Enjoy your delicious and healthy low-carb zucchini noodles with pesto!

Nutritional information per serving: Calories: 250, Fat: 18g, Carbohydrates: 8g (net 4g), Fiber: 4g, Protein: 8g

Tips:

- To remove excess moisture from the zucchini noodles, sprinkle them with 1/4 teaspoon of salt and let them sit in a colander for 10 minutes. Then, gently squeeze out any liquid before adding them to the pesto.
- If you don't have pine nuts, you can substitute with walnuts, almonds, or sunflower seeds.
- For a creamier pesto, add a tablespoon of mascarpone cheese or ricotta cheese.
- Leftovers can be stored in an airtight container in the refrigerator for up to 2 days.

Cauliflower Fried Rice

Cooking Time: 15 minutes | **Prep Time**: 10 minutes | **Total Time**: 25 minutes | **Serving Size**: 2-3

Ingredients:

- 1 head cauliflower, riced (or 4 cups frozen cauliflower rice)
- 2 tablespoons avocado oil or olive oil
- 2 eggs, beaten
- 1/2 cup diced red bell pepper
- 1/2 cup diced onion
- 2 cloves garlic, minced
- 1/4 cup chopped green onions
- 1/4 cup cooked chicken, shrimp, or tofu (optional)
- 2 tablespoons soy sauce or coconut aminos
- 1 teaspoon sesame oil
- 1/2 teaspoon Sriracha (optional)
- Salt and pepper to taste

Directions:

1. Prep the cauliflower. If using fresh cauliflower, wash and trim it, then pulse it in a food processor until it resembles rice grains. You can also use a box grater. If using frozen cauliflower rice, thaw it according to package instructions.
2. Heat the oil in a large skillet or wok over medium-high heat. Add the cauliflower rice and cook, stirring occasionally, until softened and slightly browned, about 5 minutes.
3. Push the cauliflower rice to the sides of the pan to create a well in the center. Pour in the beaten eggs and scramble until cooked through.
4. Add the red bell pepper, onion, and garlic to the pan. Stir-fry for 2-3 minutes, until the vegetables are softened but still crisp.
5. Stir in the cooked chicken, shrimp, or tofu (if using), green onions, soy sauce, sesame oil, Sriracha (if using), salt, and pepper. Cook for another minute or two, until everything is heated through.
6. Serve immediately and enjoy!

Nutritional Information per serving: Calories: 250, Carbs: 5g (net), Fat: 15g, Protein: 18g

Tips:

- You can add other vegetables to this recipe, such as broccoli, carrots, or snap peas.
- For a vegetarian option, omit the chicken, shrimp, or tofu and add 1 cup of cooked black beans or lentils.
- If you don't have Sriracha, you can use another hot sauce or red pepper flakes to taste.
- Leftovers can be stored in an airtight container in the refrigerator for up to 3 days.

Turkey Lettuce Wraps

Cooking Time: 15 minutes | **Prep Time**: 10 minutes | **Total Time**: 25 minutes | **Serving size**: 4

Ingredients:

- 1 pound ground turkey
- 1 tablespoon olive oil
- 1/2 onion, diced
- 1 red bell pepper, diced
- 2 cloves garlic, minced
- 1 tablespoon grated ginger
- 2 tablespoons soy sauce
- 1 tablespoon rice vinegar
- 1 tablespoon sriracha
- 1/2 teaspoon lime juice
- 1/4 cup chopped cilantro
- 12 butter lettuce leaves

Directions:

1. Heat olive oil in a large skillet over medium heat. Add the ground turkey and cook until browned, breaking it up with a spoon. Drain any excess fat.

2. Add the onion, bell pepper, garlic, and ginger to the skillet. Cook for 5-7 minutes, or until the vegetables are softened.

3. Stir in the soy sauce, rice vinegar, sriracha, and lime juice. Bring to a simmer and cook for 2-3 minutes, or until slightly thickened.

4. Remove from heat and stir in the cilantro.

5. Place a lettuce leaf on a plate and top with some of the turkey mixture. Enjoy immediately.

Nutritional Information per serving: Calories: 350, Fat: 15g, Carbohydrates: 5g (net carbs), Fiber: 2g, Protein: 30g

Tips:

- For a spicier wrap, add additional sriracha or a pinch of red pepper flakes.
- You can substitute ground chicken or beef for the ground turkey.
- If you don't have butter lettuce, you can use romaine or iceberg lettuce.
- Serve with additional toppings like chopped peanuts, sliced avocado, or crumbled cheese.

Eggplant Parmesan

Cooking Time: 25 minutes | **Prep Time**: 15 minutes | **Total Time**: 40 minutes | **Serving Size**: 2

Ingredients:

- 1 medium eggplant, thinly sliced
- 1 tablespoon olive oil
- 1/2 teaspoon Italian seasoning
- 1/4 teaspoon salt
- 1/4 teaspoon black pepper
- 1/2 cup marinara sauce (sugar-free preferred)
- 1/2 cup shredded mozzarella cheese
- 1/4 cup grated Parmesan cheese
- Fresh basil, for garnish (optional)

Directions:

1. Preheat oven to 400°F (200°C). Line a baking sheet with parchment paper.

2. Toss eggplant slices with olive oil, Italian seasoning, salt, and pepper. Arrange in a single layer on the prepared baking sheet.

3. Bake for 20-25 minutes, flipping halfway through, until eggplant is tender and slightly browned.

4. Spread half of the marinara sauce over the bottom of a baking dish. Top with half of the eggplant slices, then remaining marinara sauce, mozzarella cheese, and Parmesan cheese.

5. Bake for an additional 5-7 minutes, or until cheese is melted and bubbly.

6. Garnish with fresh basil, if desired, and serve immediately.

Nutritional Information per serving: Calories: 350, Fat: 20g, Carbohydrates: 8g (net carbs), Protein: 30g

Tips:

- To save time, use pre-sliced eggplant, but be sure to pat it dry with paper towels to remove excess moisture.
- If you prefer a crispier eggplant, sprinkle the slices with a pinch of cornstarch or almond flour before baking.
- For a richer flavor, add a dollop of ricotta cheese to each layer before adding the mozzarella.
- Feel free to customize the recipe with your favorite herbs and spices.

Salmon and Asparagus Foil Packets

Cooking Time: 15-20 minutes | **Prep Time**: 10 minutes | **Total Time**: 25-30 minutes | **Serving Size**: 1

Ingredients:

- 4 salmon fillets (4-6 oz each), skin on or off
- 1 pound asparagus, trimmed and cut into 1-inch pieces
- 1/4 cup olive oil
- 2 tablespoons lemon juice
- 2 cloves garlic, minced
- 1/2 teaspoon dried thyme
- Salt and pepper to taste

Directions:

1. Preheat oven to 400°F (200°C).

2. Tear off four squares of aluminum foil large enough to enclose the salmon fillets.

3. Place one salmon fillet in the center of each foil square. Top with asparagus, drizzle with olive oil, lemon juice, and sprinkle with garlic, thyme, salt, and pepper.

4. Fold the foil up over the salmon and asparagus, crimping the edges to seal.

5. Place the foil packets on a baking sheet.

6. Bake for 15-20 minutes, or until the salmon is cooked through and the asparagus is tender.

7. Carefully open the foil packets and serve immediately.

Nutritional Information per serving: Calories: 350, Fat: 25g, Carbohydrates: 5g (net), Protein: 35g, Fiber: 2g

Tips:

- You can add other vegetables to the packets, such as zucchini, bell peppers, or onions.
- If you like your salmon a little crispy, you can broil the packets for a minute or two after baking.
- To make this recipe ahead of time, assemble the packets and refrigerate them for up to 24 hours before baking.
- Serve these packets with a side of low-carb rice or quinoa, or a simple salad.

Cabbage and Beef Stir-Fry

Prep Time: 10 minutes | **Cooking Time**: 15 minutes | **Total Time**: 25 minutes | **Servings**: 2

Ingredients:

- 1 tablespoon avocado oil
- 1/2 pound ground beef (90% lean or higher)
- 1/2 head green cabbage, thinly sliced
- 1 red bell pepper, thinly sliced
- 1 onion, thinly sliced
- 2 cloves garlic, minced
- 1 tablespoon grated ginger
- 1/4 cup low-sodium chicken broth
- 2 tablespoons soy sauce
- 1 tablespoon rice vinegar
- 1 teaspoon sesame oil
- 1/2 teaspoon red pepper flakes (optional)
- Salt and pepper to taste
- Chopped green onions, for garnish
- Sesame seeds, for garnish (optional)

Directions:
1. Heat avocado oil in a large skillet or wok over medium-high heat. Add the ground beef and cook until browned, breaking it up with a spoon. Drain any excess fat.
2. Add the cabbage, bell pepper, and onion to the skillet and stir-fry for 3-4 minutes, or until the vegetables are slightly softened.
3. Add the garlic and ginger and cook for 30 seconds until fragrant.
4. In a small bowl, whisk together the chicken broth, soy sauce, rice vinegar, sesame oil, and red pepper flakes (if using). Pour the sauce into the skillet and stir to combine.
5. Cook for 1-2 minutes, or until the sauce is thickened slightly. Season with salt and pepper to taste.
6. Garnish with chopped green onions and sesame seeds (if using) and serve immediately.

Nutritional Information per serving: Calories: 350, Fat: 15g, Carbohydrates: 5g (net carbs), Fiber: 3g, Protein: 30g

Tips:

- Serve this stir-fry over a bed of cauliflower rice or shredded romaine lettuce for extra fiber and low-carb goodness.
- You can also use other low-carb vegetables in this recipe, such as broccoli, zucchini, or snap peas.
- If you don't have ground beef, you can use chicken, pork, or shrimp instead.
- To make this recipe even more flavorful, marinate the meat in soy sauce, rice vinegar, and sesame oil for 30 minutes before cooking.

Cauliflower Crust Pizza

Prep Time: 15 minutes | **Cook Time**: 35 minutes | **Total Time**: 50 minutes | **Servings**: 2

Ingredients:

- 1 head cauliflower, grated
- 1/2 cup mozzarella cheese, shredded
- 1/4 cup parmesan cheese, shredded
- 1 egg, beaten
- 1 teaspoon Italian seasoning
- 1/2 teaspoon garlic powder
- 1/4 teaspoon salt
- 1/4 teaspoon black pepper
- Pizza sauce (low-carb or sugar-free)
- Your favorite toppings (such as pepperoni, sausage, mushrooms, onions, peppers, etc.)

Directions:

1. Preheat oven to 400°F (200°C). Line a baking sheet with parchment paper.
2. Grate the cauliflower using a food processor or box grater. Pulse until it resembles rice. Place the grated cauliflower in a microwave-safe bowl and microwave for 3-4 minutes, or until softened.
3. Transfer the cauliflower to a clean kitchen towel or nut milk bag and squeeze out as much moisture as possible. The drier the cauliflower, the crispier the crust will be.
4. In a large bowl, combine the drained cauliflower, mozzarella cheese, parmesan cheese, egg, Italian seasoning, garlic powder, salt, and pepper. Mix well until everything is evenly combined.
5. Transfer the cauliflower mixture to the prepared baking sheet and spread it into an even circle, about 12 inches in diameter. Press down to form a compact crust.
6. Bake for 20-25 minutes, or until the crust is golden brown and firm to the touch.
7. Remove the crust from the oven and spread with your desired amount of pizza sauce. Top with your favorite toppings.
8. Bake for an additional 10-15 minutes, or until the cheese is melted and bubbly and the toppings are cooked through.
9. Let the pizza cool for a few minutes before slicing and serving. Enjoy your delicious and healthy low-carb cauliflower crust pizza!

Nutritional Information per serving: Calories: 350, Fat: 20g, Carbohydrates: 10g (net carbs 5g), Protein: 25g

Tips:
- For a thicker crust, pre-bake the cauliflower rice for 10 minutes before adding the other ingredients.
- You can also use pre-riced cauliflower to save time.
- Get creative with your toppings! Try different low-carb vegetables, meats, and cheeses to find your perfect combination.
- Leftovers can be stored in the refrigerator for up to 3 days.

Shrimp Avocado Salad

Cooking Time: 10 minutes | **Prep Time**: 15 minutes | **Total Time**: 25 minutes | **Serving Size**: 1 large salad

Ingredients:

- 1 pound raw shrimp, peeled and deveined (or 12 oz cooked shrimp)
- 1 ripe avocado, pitted and diced
- 1 cucumber, thinly sliced
- 1/2 red onion, thinly sliced
- 1/4 cup cherry tomatoes, halved
- 1/4 cup fresh cilantro, chopped
- 2 tablespoons olive oil
- 1 tablespoon fresh lime juice
- 1/2 teaspoon cumin
- 1/4 teaspoon chili powder
- Salt and pepper to taste

Directions:

1. If using raw shrimp, cook them in boiling water for 3-4 minutes, or until opaque and cooked through. Drain and cool slightly.

2. In a large bowl, combine the shrimp, avocado, cucumber, red onion, and cherry tomatoes.

3. In a separate small bowl, whisk together the olive oil, lime juice, cumin, chili powder, salt, and pepper.

4. Pour the dressing over the salad and toss to coat.

5. Garnish with fresh cilantro and serve immediately.

Nutritional Information per serving: Calories: 350, Fat: 20g (mostly healthy fats), Protein: 30g, Carbohydrates: 5g (net carbs), Fiber: 2g

Tips:

- For a spicier salad, add a pinch of cayenne pepper to the dressing.
- If you don't have fresh cilantro, you can substitute parsley or dill.
- You can also add other low-carb vegetables to the salad, such as chopped bell peppers, zucchini, or spinach.
- Serve the salad on a bed of romaine lettuce or baby spinach for added nutrients.

Greek Salad with Grilled Chicken

Cooking Time: 8-10 minutes | **Prep Time**: 15 minutes | **Total Time**: 25 minutes | **Serving Size**: 1 large salad

Ingredients:

For the Chicken:
- 1 boneless, skinless chicken breast (150g)
- 1 tablespoon olive oil
- 1/2 teaspoon dried oregano
- 1/4 teaspoon garlic powder
- Salt and pepper to taste

For the Salad:
- 2 cups romaine lettuce, chopped
- 1 cucumber, sliced
- 1/2 red onion, thinly sliced
- 1/2 cup cherry tomatoes, halved
- 1/4 cup Kalamata olives, pitted and halved
- 1/4 cup crumbled feta cheese

For the Dressing:
- 2 tablespoons olive oil
- 1 tablespoon lemon juice
- 1 teaspoon red wine vinegar
- 1/2 teaspoon dried oregano
- 1/4 teaspoon garlic powder
- Pinch of salt and pepper

Directions:

1. Marinate the chicken: In a small bowl, combine olive oil, oregano, garlic powder, salt, and pepper. Place the chicken in the marinade and toss to coat. Let sit for at least 15 minutes, or up to 30 minutes.
2. Grill the chicken: Preheat your grill or grill pan to medium-high heat. Grill the chicken for 4-5 minutes per side, or until cooked through. Remove from heat and let cool slightly.
3. Prepare the salad: In a large bowl, combine romaine lettuce, cucumber, red onion, cherry tomatoes, and Kalamata olives.
4. Make the dressing: In a small jar or bowl, whisk together olive oil, lemon juice, red wine vinegar, oregano, garlic powder, salt, and pepper.
5. Assemble the salad: Slice the grilled chicken and add it to the salad bowl. Crumble feta cheese over the top and drizzle with the dressing. Toss gently to combine.
6. Enjoy!

Nutritional Information per serving: Calories: 450, Fat: 25g (healthy fats), Carbohydrates: 10g (net carbs), Protein: 40g

Tips:

- For added flavor, marinate the chicken in the fridge for several hours or overnight.
- You can also substitute chicken thighs for breasts for a richer flavor.
- If you don't have a grill, you can cook the chicken in a grill pan or skillet over medium heat.
- Add other low-carb vegetables to the salad, such as bell peppers, zucchini, or spinach.
- For a dairy-free option, omit the feta cheese or use a vegan alternative.

Crispy Baked Zucchini Fries

Prep Time: 15 minutes |**Cook Time**: 20-25 minutes |**Total Time**: 40 minutes |**Serving Size**: 2

Ingredients:

- 2 medium zucchinis
- 1 egg, beaten
- 1/2 cup almond flour
- 1/4 cup grated Parmesan cheese
- 1 teaspoon dried oregano
- 1/2 teaspoon garlic powder
- 1/4 teaspoon onion powder
- Salt and pepper to taste

Instructions:

1. Preheat oven to 425°F (220°C). Line a baking sheet with parchment paper.
2. Wash and dry the zucchinis. Cut them into thin strips, about 1/4-inch thick and 3-4 inches long.
3. In a shallow bowl, whisk together the beaten egg. In another bowl, combine the almond flour, Parmesan cheese, oregano, garlic powder, onion powder, salt, and pepper.
4. Dip each zucchini strip in the egg wash, then toss it in the almond flour mixture to coat evenly. Place the coated fries on the prepared baking sheet in a single layer, making sure they don't touch.
5. Bake for 20-25 minutes, or until golden brown and crispy. Flip the fries halfway through baking for even cooking.

Nutritional Information per serving: Calories: 150, Fat: 8g, Carbohydrates: 5g (3g net carbs), Fiber: 2g, Protein: 4g

Tips:

- For extra flavor, you can sprinkle the fries with additional spices like paprika, chili powder, or cayenne pepper before baking.
- If you don't have almond flour, you can use coconut flour or pork rind crumbs as a substitute.
- If your zucchini fries are not getting crispy enough, you can try preheating the baking sheet before adding the fries.
- These fries are best served hot and fresh, but they can also be stored in an airtight container in the refrigerator for up to 2 days. Reheat them in the oven or air fryer before serving.

Cucumber Bites

Cooking Time: None |**Prep Time**: 10 minutes |**Total Time**: 10 minutes |**Serving Size**: 12

Ingredients:

- 1 medium cucumber
- 4 oz cream cheese, softened
- 2 tbsp mayonnaise or Greek yogurt
- 1 tbsp chopped fresh herbs (dill, chives, parsley, or your choice)
- 1/2 tsp lemon juice
- 1/4 tsp garlic powder
- Salt and pepper to taste
- Optional toppings: diced red bell pepper, crumbled feta cheese, chopped olives, everything bagel seasoning, smoked paprika

Directions:

1. Wash and dry the cucumber. Slice it into 1/2-inch rounds. Using a melon baller or a small spoon, scoop out the seeds from the center of each slice, creating little cups.
2. In a small bowl, combine the softened cream cheese, mayonnaise or Greek yogurt, herbs, lemon juice, garlic powder, salt, and pepper. Mix until smooth and creamy.
3. Fill each cucumber cup with the cream cheese mixture. Top with your desired toppings.
4. Refrigerate for at least 30 minutes before serving. This allows the flavors to meld and the cucumber to become slightly softened.

Nutritional Information per serving: Calories: 30-40, Carbohydrates: 1-2 g, Fat: 2-3 g, Protein: 1-2 g

Tips:

- For a richer flavor, use full-fat cream cheese.
- If you don't have fresh herbs, you can use 1/2 teaspoon of dried herbs.
- Get creative with your toppings! Chopped nuts, seeds, or crumbled bacon are all delicious options.
- These bites can be made ahead of time and stored in the refrigerator for up to 2 days.

Deviled Eggs

Cooking Time: 12 minutes |**Prep Time**: 15 minutes |**Total Time**: 27 minutes |**Serving Size**: 12

Ingredients:

- 6 large eggs
- 1/4 cup mayonnaise (avocado oil mayo preferred)
- 2 tablespoons Dijon mustard
- 1 tablespoon apple cider vinegar
- 1/2 teaspoon paprika
- 1/4 teaspoon salt
- 1/4 teaspoon black pepper
- Chives or parsley, for garnish (optional)

Directions:

1. Hard-boil the eggs: Place the eggs in a saucepan and cover them with cold water. Bring to a boil over high heat, then immediately remove from heat and cover. Let the eggs sit for 12 minutes, then drain and cool under cold running water. Peel the eggs carefully.
2. Cut and separate the eggs: Slice each egg in half lengthwise. Carefully scoop out the yolks and place them in a bowl. Set the empty egg whites aside on a serving platter.
3. Mash the yolks: Mash the yolks with a fork until smooth.
4. Mix the filling: Add the mayonnaise, Dijon mustard, apple cider vinegar, paprika, salt, and pepper to the mashed yolks. Mix well until smooth and creamy.
5. Fill the eggs: Using a spoon or piping bag, pipe or scoop the filling into the egg white halves.
6. Chill and garnish: Cover the eggs and refrigerate for at least 30 minutes, this allows the flavors to meld and the filling to firm up. Garnish with chives or parsley before serving (optional).

Nutritional Information per serving: Calories: 100, Fat: 7g, Carbs: 0.5g, Protein: 6g, Fiber: 0g

Tips:

- For a richer flavor, add 1/4 of a ripe avocado to the yolk mixture.
- If you prefer a spicier kick, add a pinch of cayenne pepper to the filling.
- Substitute sour cream for some or all of the mayonnaise for a tangier filling.
- To make peeling the eggs easier, add a teaspoon of baking soda to the water when boiling them.
- Store leftover deviled eggs in an airtight container in the refrigerator for up to 3 days.

Baked Buffalo Cauliflower Bites

Cooking Time: 20-25 minutes |**Prep Time**: 10 minutes |**Total Time**: 30 minutes |**Serving Size**: 12

Ingredients:

- 1 head cauliflower, cut into bite-sized florets
- 1/4 cup almond flour
- 1/4 teaspoon garlic powder
- 1/4 teaspoon onion powder
- 1/4 teaspoon smoked paprika
- 1/8 teaspoon salt
- 1/8 teaspoon black pepper
- 1/4 cup hot sauce
- 1 tablespoon melted butter
- 1 tablespoon olive oil
- Blue cheese dressing or ranch dressing, for dipping (optional)

Directions:

1. Preheat oven to 425°F (220°C). Line a baking sheet with parchment paper.
2. In a medium bowl, whisk together almond flour, garlic powder, onion powder, paprika, salt, and pepper.
3. Add cauliflower florets to the bowl and toss to coat evenly with the dry mixture.
4. In a separate bowl, whisk together hot sauce, melted butter, and olive oil.
5. Pour the wet mixture over the coated cauliflower florets and toss to coat.
6. Spread the cauliflower florets in a single layer on the prepared baking sheet.
7. Bake for 20-25 minutes, or until the cauliflower is tender and crispy.
8. Serve immediately with blue cheese dressing or ranch dressing, if desired.

Nutritional Information per serving: Calories: 150, Fat: 8g, Carbs: 5g (net), Protein: 5g, Fiber: 3g

Tips:

- For extra crispy cauliflower, broil for the last minute or two of baking.
- If you don't have almond flour, you can use chickpea flour or a mixture of ground flaxseed and pork rind crumbs.
- Add a teaspoon of chopped celery seed to the buffalo sauce for a more traditional buffalo wing flavor.
- These bites can be stored in an airtight container in the refrigerator for up to 3 days.

Cheese Crisps

Prep Time: 5 minutes |**Cooking Time**: 10-12 minutes |**Total Time**: 15-17 minutes |**Serving Size**: Makes about 20 crisps

Ingredients:

- 1 cup shredded cheddar cheese (sharp or mild)
- 1/4 cup grated Parmesan cheese
- 1/4 teaspoon dried oregano
- 1/4 teaspoon paprika
- Pinch of cayenne pepper (optional)
- Parchment paper

Instructions:

- Preheat oven to 375°F (190°C). Line a baking sheet with parchment paper.
- In a medium bowl, combine the cheddar cheese, Parmesan cheese, oregano, paprika, and cayenne pepper (if using). Mix well.
- Drop heaping tablespoons of the cheese mixture onto the prepared baking sheet, leaving space between each for spreading.
- Bake for 10-12 minutes, or until golden brown and crispy around the edges.
- Let cool on the baking sheet for a few minutes before serving. Enjoy warm or at room temperature.

Nutritional Information per crisp: Calories: 50, Fat: 4g, Carbs: 0.5g, Protein: 4g

Tips:

- For a variety of flavors, try using different types of cheese, such as Gruyere, Monterey Jack, or pepper jack.
- Add a sprinkle of your favorite herbs or spices, such as rosemary, thyme, or garlic powder.
- Serve with your favorite low-carb dips, such as guacamole, salsa, or sour cream.
- Store leftover crisps in an airtight container at room temperature for up to 3 days.

Stuffed Mushrooms

Cooking Time: 20-25 minutes |**Prep Time**: 15 minutes |**Total Time**: 40 minutes |**Serving Size**: 10

Ingredients:

- 12 large portobello mushrooms (or large white button mushrooms)
- 1 tablespoon olive oil
- 1/2 onion, finely chopped
- 2 cloves garlic, minced
- 4 ounces ground sausage (optional)
- 4 ounces cream cheese, softened
- 1/2 cup shredded cheddar cheese
- 1/4 cup chopped fresh parsley
- Salt and pepper to taste

Directions:

1. Preheat oven to 375°F (190°C).
2. Gently clean the mushrooms with a damp paper towel. Remove the stems and finely chop them. Set the caps aside.
3. In a medium skillet over medium heat, heat olive oil. Add the onion and cook until softened, about 5 minutes. Add the garlic and cook for an additional minute.
4. If using sausage, add it to the skillet and cook until browned. Drain any excess fat.
5. In a bowl, combine the cream cheese, cheddar cheese, parsley, salt, and pepper. Stir in the cooked onion, garlic, and sausage (if using).
6. Fill each mushroom cap with the mixture.
7. Arrange the stuffed mushrooms on a baking sheet.
8. Bake for 20-25 minutes, or until the mushrooms are tender and the filling is bubbly.
9. Serve immediately.

Nutritional Information per serving: Calories: 150, Fat: 10g, Carbs: 4g (net), Protein: 8g

Tips:

- For a vegetarian option, omit the sausage.
- You can also use other types of cheese, such as mozzarella or Gruyère.
- Add a sprinkle of chopped nuts or breadcrumbs for a bit of crunch.
- Top with a dollop of Greek yogurt or sour cream for added richness.

Guacamole with Veggie Sticks

Prep Time: 10 minutes |**Cooking Time**: 0 minutes |**Total Time**: 10 minutes |**Serving Size**: 4-6 servings

Ingredients:

- 2 ripe avocados
- 1/2 lime, juiced
- 1/4 red onion, finely chopped
- 1 small tomato, finely chopped
- 1/4 cup fresh cilantro, chopped
- Salt and pepper to taste

Directions:

1. Prep the avocados: Cut the avocados in half and remove the pits. Scoop out the flesh into a bowl.
2. Mash the avocados: Using a fork or a potato masher, mash the avocado flesh to your desired consistency. Some people prefer a chunky guacamole, while others prefer it smooth.
3. Add the lime juice, red onion, tomato, and cilantro: Stir in the lime juice, red onion, tomato, and cilantro. Season with salt and pepper to taste.
4. Taste and adjust: Taste the guacamole and adjust the seasonings as needed. If you want it spicier, add a finely chopped jalapeño pepper. For a more herbaceous flavor, add a tablespoon of chopped fresh parsley. You can also add a tablespoon of olive oil for a richer flavor.
5. Serve with veggie sticks: Cut up your favorite low-carb vegetables into sticks, such as celery, cucumber, bell peppers, and carrots. Serve the guacamole with the veggie sticks.

Nutritional Information per Serving: Calories: 149, Fat: 13g, Carbohydrates: 4g (2g fiber), Protein: 2g

Tips:

- For the best flavor, use ripe avocados. They should be slightly soft to the touch but not mushy.
- If you're not serving the guacamole right away, store it in an airtight container in the refrigerator. To prevent browning, you can press a piece of plastic wrap directly onto the surface of the guacamole.
- This guacamole recipe is naturally low in carbs and can be enjoyed on a keto diet. However, be sure to check the carb content of your veggie sticks, as some vegetables, such as potatoes and corn, are higher in carbs.

Crispy Bacon-Wrapped Asparagus

Cooking Time: 15-20 minutes |**Prep Time**: 10 minutes |**Total Time**: 25-30 minutes |**Serving Size**: 12

Ingredients:

- 1 bundle asparagus (12-15 spears)
- 12 slices bacon, cut in half
- 1 tablespoon olive oil
- 1/2 teaspoon salt
- 1/4 teaspoon black pepper

Directions:

1. Preheat oven to 400°F (200°C). Line a baking sheet with parchment paper.
2. Trim the woody ends of the asparagus spears.
3. Brush each asparagus spear with olive oil. Sprinkle with salt and pepper.
4. Wrap each asparagus spear with half a slice of bacon, starting at the thicker end and spiraling upwards. Secure with a toothpick if desired.
5. Arrange the bacon-wrapped asparagus in a single layer on the prepared baking sheet.
6. Bake for 15-20 minutes, or until the bacon is crispy and the asparagus is tender-crisp.
7. Let cool slightly before serving.

Nutritional Information per serving: Calories: 70, Fat: 5g, Carbohydrates: 1g (net), Protein: 5g

Tips:

- For extra flavor, drizzle the asparagus with balsamic vinegar or a squeeze of lemon juice before serving.
- You can also grill the bacon-wrapped asparagus for a smoky flavor.
- To make this recipe ahead of time, prepare the asparagus as instructed and then refrigerate for up to 24 hours. When ready to cook, bake from a cold start for an additional 5-10 minutes.

Antipasto Skewers

Prep Time: 10 minutes |**Cooking Time**: 0 minutes |**Total Time**: 10 minutes |**Servings**: 12

Ingredients:

- 12 cherry tomatoes
- 1/4 cup sliced roasted red peppers
- 1/2 cup marinated artichoke hearts, drained and quartered
- 12 bocconcini balls (small mozzarella balls)
- 12 green olives, pitted
- 12 fresh basil leaves
- 12 slices Genoa salami
- 2 tablespoons balsamic vinegar

Directions:

1. Assemble the skewers: Thread a cherry tomato, a slice of roasted red pepper, an artichoke heart quarter, a bocconcini ball, an olive, and a basil leaf onto each skewer. Wrap a slice of salami around the bottom of each skewer to secure.
2. Drizzle with balsamic vinegar: Place the skewers on a plate and drizzle with balsamic vinegar. Serve immediately.

Nutritional Information per skewer: Calories: 150, Fat: 10g, Carbohydrates: 2g (net), Protein: 12g

Tips:
- You can customize these skewers to your liking. Try using different types of olives, cheeses, or meats.
- For a smoky flavor, grill the cherry tomatoes before threading them onto the skewers.
- If you don't have balsamic vinegar, you can use another low-carb vinegar, such as apple cider vinegar or red wine vinegar.
- Make these skewers ahead of time and store them in the refrigerator for up to 24 hours.

Cauliflower Hummus with Veggie Dippers

Cooking Time: 20 minutes |**Prep Time**: 10 minutes |**Total Time**: 30 minutes |**Serving Size**: 6

Ingredients:
- 1 head cauliflower, trimmed and cut into florets
- 1/4 cup tahini
- 2 tablespoons olive oil
- 2 cloves garlic, minced
- 1/4 cup lemon juice
- 1/4 cup water
- 1/2 teaspoon dried cumin
- 1/4 teaspoon smoked paprika
- Salt and pepper to taste

For the Veggie Dippers:
- Carrot sticks
- Cucumber sticks
- Bell pepper slices
- Celery sticks
- Broccoli florets
- Cherry tomatoes

Directions:
1. Preheat oven to 400°F (200°C). Spread the cauliflower florets on a baking sheet and drizzle with olive oil. Roast for 20-25 minutes, or until tender and lightly browned.
2. While the cauliflower is roasting, prepare the hummus. In a food processor, combine the tahini, olive oil, garlic, lemon juice, water, cumin, paprika, salt, and pepper. Blend until smooth.
3. Add the roasted cauliflower to the food processor and blend until creamy, scraping down the sides as needed. Adjust the consistency with additional water if desired.
4. Transfer the hummus to a serving bowl and garnish with a drizzle of olive oil, paprika, and a sprinkle of chopped fresh parsley (optional).
5. Arrange the veggie dippers around the hummus and serve with additional lemon wedges, if desired.

Nutritional Information per Serving: Calories: 150, Fat: 8g, Carbohydrates: 5g (2g net carbs), Fiber: 3g, Protein: 5g

Tips:

- For a smoother hummus, you can peel the cauliflower before roasting.
- If you don't have tahini, you can substitute almond butter or cashew butter.
- Feel free to adjust the spices to your taste. You can also add other herbs and spices, such as coriander, oregano, or chili flakes.
- This hummus can be stored in an airtight container in the refrigerator for up to 3 days.

Broccoli Cheddar Soup

Prep Time: 10 minutes |**Cook Time**: 20 minutes |**Total Time**: 30 minutes |**Servings**: 4

Ingredients:

- 1 tablespoon butter
- 1 onion, chopped
- 2 cloves garlic, minced
- 4 cups chicken broth (low-sodium)
- 2 cups broccoli florets
- 1 cup heavy cream
- 4 ounces cheddar cheese, shredded
- Salt and pepper to taste
- Optional garnishes: chopped chives, crumbled bacon, or red pepper flakes

Directions:

1. Melt the butter in a large pot over medium heat. Add the onion and cook until softened, about 5 minutes.
2. Add the garlic and cook for 30 seconds, until fragrant.
3. Stir in the chicken broth and broccoli florets. Bring to a boil, then reduce heat to low and simmer for 15-20 minutes, or until the broccoli is tender.
4. While the soup is simmering, heat the heavy cream in a small saucepan over medium heat until warmed through. Do not boil.
5. Once the broccoli is tender, use an immersion blender or blender to puree the soup until smooth.
6. Stir in the warmed heavy cream and cheddar cheese. Season with salt and pepper to taste.
7. Serve immediately, garnished with chopped chives, crumbled bacon, or red pepper flakes, if desired.

Nutritional Information per Serving: Calories: 340, Fat: 24g, Carbohydrates: 4g (net), Protein: 22g, Fiber: 3g

Tips:

- For a thicker soup, use less broth or simmer for a longer time.
- You can also add other low-carb vegetables to the soup, such as cauliflower, zucchini, or bell peppers.
- If you don't have an immersion blender, you can transfer the soup to a blender in batches to puree it.
- To make this soup dairy-free, use vegetable broth and vegan cheese.

Chicken Zoodle Soup

Cooking time: 15 minutes |**Prep time**: 10 minutes |**Total time**: 25 minutes |**Serving size**: 4

Ingredients:

- 1 tablespoon olive oil
- 1/2 onion, diced
- 2 carrots, peeled and diced
- 2 celery stalks, diced
- 2 cloves garlic, minced
- 4 cups chicken broth
- 1 pound boneless, skinless chicken breasts, cooked and shredded
- 3 medium zucchini, spiralized
- 1/2 teaspoon dried thyme
- Salt and pepper to taste
- Chopped fresh parsley, for garnish (optional)

Instructions:

1. Heat olive oil in a large pot over medium heat. Add onion, carrots, and celery and cook until softened, about 5 minutes.
2. Add garlic and cook for 30 seconds more.
3. Pour in chicken broth and bring to a boil.
4. Reduce heat to simmer and add cooked chicken, zucchini noodles, and thyme.
5. Simmer for 5-10 minutes, or until zucchini noodles are tender-crisp.
6. Season with salt and pepper to taste.
7. Serve hot, garnished with chopped parsley if desired.

Nutritional information per serving: Calories: 200, Fat: 8g, Protein: 25g, Carbs: 5g (net)

Tips:

- You can use leftover rotisserie chicken for this recipe.
- If you don't have a spiralizer, you can use a julienne peeler or thinly slice the zucchini with a knife.
- For a thicker soup, use a potato masher to partially mash some of the zucchini noodles before adding them to the pot.
- Add other low-carb vegetables to the soup, such as broccoli, green beans, or mushrooms.
- Serve this soup with a side of low-carb bread or crackers for a complete meal.

Tomato Basil Soup

Prep Time: 10 minutes **Cooking Time**: 25 minutes |**Total Time**: 35 minutes |**Servings**: 4

Ingredients:

- 2 tablespoons olive oil
- 1 medium onion, diced
- 2 cloves garlic, minced
- 28 ounces canned crushed tomatoes (preferably San Marzano)
- 4 cups chicken broth or vegetable broth
- 1/2 cup chopped fresh basil
- 1/2 teaspoon dried oregano
- Salt and pepper to taste
- Optional toppings: Heavy cream, Parmesan cheese, fresh basil leaves

Instructions:

1. Heat olive oil in a large pot or Dutch oven over medium heat. Add the onion and cook until softened, about 5 minutes.
2. Add the garlic and cook for another minute until fragrant.
3. Add the crushed tomatoes, chicken broth, oregano, salt, and pepper. Bring to a boil, then reduce heat and simmer for 20 minutes.
4. Stir in the chopped basil and simmer for another 5 minutes.
5. Use an immersion blender or transfer the soup to a blender and puree until smooth.
6. Return the soup to the pot and warm through if necessary.
7. Serve hot, topped with a swirl of heavy cream, Parmesan cheese, and fresh basil leaves, if desired.

Nutritional Information per Serving: Calories: 150, Fat: 8g, Carbohydrates: 6g (3g net carbs), Protein: 5g, Fiber: 3g

Tips:

- For a thicker soup, use a potato masher or immersion blender to leave some of the tomatoes chunky.
- You can also add other vegetables to this soup, such as bell peppers, zucchini, or spinach.
- If you don't have fresh basil, you can use 1 tablespoon of dried basil instead.
- This soup can be stored in the refrigerator for up to 3 days.

Cauliflower Soup

Prep time: 15 minutes |**Cooking time**: 30 minutes |**Total time**: 45 minutes |**Serving size**: 4

Ingredients:

- 1 head cauliflower, cut into florets
- 1 tablespoon olive oil
- 1/2 teaspoon salt
- 1/4 teaspoon black pepper
- 1 onion, chopped
- 2 cloves garlic, minced
- 4 cups chicken broth or vegetable broth
- 1 cup unsweetened almond milk
- 1/2 cup heavy cream (optional)
- 1/4 cup grated Parmesan cheese
- Fresh herbs (optional, for garnish)

Directions:

1. Preheat oven to 400°F (200°C). Toss cauliflower florets with olive oil, salt, and pepper. Spread on a baking sheet and roast for 20-25 minutes, until tender and lightly browned.
2. While cauliflower is roasting, heat remaining olive oil in a large pot over medium heat. Add onion and cook until softened, about 5 minutes. Add garlic and cook for another minute, until fragrant.
3. Pour in broth and almond milk. Bring to a simmer and add roasted cauliflower. Simmer for 10 minutes, or until cauliflower is very tender.
4. Using an immersion blender or in batches in a regular blender, puree the soup until smooth and creamy. Stir in heavy cream (if using) and Parmesan cheese. Season with additional salt and pepper to taste.
5. Serve hot, garnished with fresh herbs (optional).

Nutritional information per serving: Calories: 180, Fat: 13g, Carbohydrates: 4g (net carbs), Protein: 10g, Fiber: 3g

Tips:

- For a thicker soup, you can leave out some of the almond milk or puree with less liquid.
- You can also substitute coconut milk for the almond milk for a richer flavor.
- Add a protein boost by stirring in shredded chicken or cooked shrimp before serving.
- Leftovers can be stored in the refrigerator for up to 3 days.

Lemon Chicken Soup

Prep Time: 10 minutes |**Cooking Time**: 20 minutes |**Total Time**: 30 minutes |**Servings**: 4

Ingredients:

- 1 tablespoon olive oil
- 1/2 onion, diced
- 1 celery stalk, diced
- 2 cloves garlic, minced
- 4 cups chicken broth
- 1 pound boneless, skinless chicken breast, cut into bite-sized pieces
- 1 cup frozen cauliflower florets
- 1/2 teaspoon dried thyme
- Salt and pepper to taste
- 1/4 cup fresh lemon juice
- Fresh parsley, chopped (optional)

Directions:

1. Sauté the vegetables: Heat olive oil in a large pot over medium heat. Add onion and celery, and cook until softened, about 5 minutes. Stir in garlic and cook for 30 seconds more.
2. Add broth and chicken: Pour in the chicken broth and bring to a boil. Add the chicken and cauliflower florets, then reduce heat to simmer and cook for 15-20 minutes, or until chicken is cooked through.
3. Season and thicken: Stir in thyme, salt, and pepper to taste. Using an immersion blender or in batches in a blender, puree the soup until slightly thickened. This adds creaminess without extra carbs.
4. Lemony finish: Add lemon juice and taste again, adjusting seasonings as needed. Garnish with fresh parsley (optional) and serve hot.

Nutritional Information per Serving: Calories: 220, Fat: 7g, Carbohydrates: 5g (net carbs 3g), Protein: 25g, Fiber: 2g

Tips:

- For a richer flavor, add a bay leaf while simmering the soup. Discard before serving.
- If you prefer a thinner soup, add more broth or water before blending.
- Leftovers can be stored in an airtight container in the refrigerator for up to 3 days.

Greek Salad

Prep Time: 10 minutes |**Cooking Time**: 0 minutes |**Total Time**: 10 minutes |**Servings**: 2

Ingredients:

- 2 cups mixed greens (optional)
- 1 cucumber, diced
- 1/2 cup cherry tomatoes, halved
- 1/2 green bell pepper, diced
- 1/4 red onion, diced (optional)
- 1/2 cup Kalamata olives, halved
- 1/4 cup crumbled feta cheese
- 2 tablespoons olive oil
- 1 tablespoon lemon juice
- 1/2 teaspoon dried oregano
- 1/4 teaspoon salt
- 1/4 teaspoon black pepper

Directions:

1. Prep the vegetables: Wash and chop the cucumber, tomatoes, bell pepper, and red onion (if using).
2. Assemble the salad: In a large bowl, combine the mixed greens (if using), chopped vegetables, olives, and feta cheese.
3. Make the dressing: In a small bowl, whisk together the olive oil, lemon juice, oregano, salt, and pepper.
4. Dress the salad: Drizzle the dressing over the salad and toss to combine.
5. Serve immediately and enjoy!

Nutritional Information per serving: Calories: 320, Fat: 24g, Carbohydrates: 6g (3g net carbs), Protein: 18g, Fiber: 3g

Tips:

- For added flavor, try grilling the bell pepper or red onion before adding them to the salad.
- If you're not a fan of raw onion, you can marinate it in red wine vinegar for 15 minutes before adding it to the salad.
- Feel free to customize this recipe with your favorite low-carb vegetables. Some good options include zucchini, avocado, and artichoke hearts.
- Make a larger batch of the dressing and store it in the refrigerator for up to a week.
- This salad is perfect for a light lunch, a refreshing side dish, or a healthy snack.

Cobb Salad

Cooking Time: 20 minutes | **Prep Time**: 15 minutes | **Total Time**: 35 minutes | **Serving Size**: 2 large salads

Ingredients:

- 4 cups chopped romaine lettuce
- 1 cup shredded cooked chicken breast (grilled, baked, or rotisserie)
- 6 slices crispy bacon, crumbled
- 2 hard-boiled eggs, quartered
- 1/2 avocado, sliced
- 1/2 cup cherry tomatoes, halved
- 1/4 cup crumbled blue cheese
- 2 tablespoons olive oil
- 1 tablespoon apple cider vinegar
- 1 teaspoon Dijon mustard
- 1/2 teaspoon dried oregano
- Salt and pepper to taste

Directions:

1. Prepare the dressing: In a small bowl, whisk together olive oil, apple cider vinegar, Dijon mustard, oregano, salt, and pepper. Set aside.

2. Assemble the salad: Divide the romaine lettuce between two large bowls or plates. Top each with equal amounts of chicken, bacon, eggs, avocado, and cherry tomatoes.

3. Drizzle with dressing and crumble blue cheese over the top. Serve immediately.

Nutritional Information per Serving: Calories: 520, Carbohydrates: 5g (net), Fat: 42g, Protein: 35g

Tips:

- For added flavor, grill the chicken breasts or bacon.
- If you don't have blue cheese, you can substitute crumbled feta or goat cheese.
- Add some extra crunch with chopped celery or radishes.
- To make this salad ahead of time, store the dressing and salad ingredients separately in the refrigerator. Assemble just before serving.

Caesar Salad

Cooking Time: 10 minutes | **Prep Time**: 10 minutes | **Total Time**: 20 minutes | **Serving Size**: 1 large salad

Ingredients:

For the Salad:
- 4 cups romaine lettuce, chopped
- 1/2 cup grilled chicken breast, sliced (optional)
- 1/4 cup cherry tomatoes, halved
- 1/4 cup avocado, sliced
- 1/4 cup Parmesan cheese, shaved

For the Dressing:
- 1/4 cup mayonnaise
- 2 tablespoons sour cream
- 2 tablespoons lemon juice
- 1 tablespoon Dijon mustard
- 1 teaspoon Worcestershire sauce
- 1/2 teaspoon garlic powder
- 1/4 teaspoon anchovy paste (optional)
- Salt and pepper to taste

Directions:

1. Make the dressing: In a blender or food processor, combine all of the dressing ingredients and blend until smooth. Season with salt and pepper to taste.

2. Prepare the salad: Chop the romaine lettuce and arrange it in a large bowl. Add the chicken, tomatoes, avocado, and Parmesan cheese.

3. Toss and serve: Drizzle the dressing over the salad and toss to combine. Serve immediately.

Nutritional Information per serving: Calories: 350, Fat: 25g, Carbohydrates: 5g (net), Protein: 30g

Tips:

- For a vegan option, omit the chicken and Parmesan cheese. You can also use a vegan mayonnaise and sour cream.
- To make the salad ahead of time, store the dressing and salad ingredients separately in the refrigerator. Assemble the salad just before serving.
- If you don't have anchovy paste, you can substitute with a few anchovy fillets, minced.

Spinach Salad with Bacon and Eggs

Cooking time: 15 minutes | **Prep time**: 10 minutes | **Total time**: 25 minutes | **Serving size**: 2

Ingredients:

- 5 oz baby spinach
- 4 slices bacon, cooked and crumbled
- 2 hard-boiled eggs, sliced
- 1/2 avocado, diced
- 1/4 cup cherry tomatoes, halved
- 1/4 red onion, thinly sliced (optional)
- 2 tablespoons olive oil
- 2 tablespoons apple cider vinegar
- 1 teaspoon Dijon mustard
- Salt and pepper to taste

Directions:

1. In a large bowl, combine the spinach, bacon, eggs, avocado, tomatoes, and red onion (if using).

2. In a small bowl, whisk together the olive oil, apple cider vinegar, Dijon mustard, salt, and pepper.

3. Pour the dressing over the salad and toss to coat.

4. Serve immediately.

Nutritional information per serving: Calories: 420, Fat: 30g, Carbohydrates: 3g (net), Protein: 25g, Fiber: 2g

Tips:

- For a warmer salad, cook the bacon until crispy and then crumble it over the top of the salad.
- You can add other low-carb vegetables to this salad, such as cucumber, bell peppers, or mushrooms.
- If you don't have apple cider vinegar, you can use white vinegar or lemon juice.
- This salad can be stored in the refrigerator for up to 2 days.

Caprese Salad

Cooking Time: None | **Prep Time**: 10 minutes | **Total Time**: 10 minutes | **Serving Size**: 1

Ingredients:

- 2 large ripe tomatoes, sliced into ½ inch rounds
- 6 ounces fresh mozzarella cheese, sliced into ½ inch rounds
- ½ avocado, sliced into ½ inch rounds
- ½ cup baby spinach or arugula
- 1/4 cup fresh basil leaves
- 2 tablespoons olive oil
- 1 tablespoon balsamic vinegar reduction
- ½ teaspoon dried oregano
- Salt and pepper to taste

Directions:

1. Assemble the salad on a plate or in a shallow bowl. Layer the tomato slices, mozzarella slices, avocado slices, and baby spinach/arugula.

2. Tear or chiffonade the basil leaves and sprinkle them over the salad.

3. Drizzle with olive oil and balsamic reduction.

4. Sprinkle with dried oregano and season with salt and pepper to taste.

5. Enjoy immediately!

Nutritional Information per serving: Calories: 240, Carbs: 6g (net), Fat: 18g, Protein: 14g, Fiber: 2g

Tips:

- For a richer flavor, grill the tomato slices briefly before assembling the salad.
- Substitute bocconcini balls for the mozzarella slices for a fun finger food presentation.
- Add a sprinkle of chopped red onion or Kalamata olives for a bit of bite.
- If you don't have balsamic reduction, you can use regular balsamic vinegar mixed with a teaspoon of sweetener (optional).
- Adjust the amount of cheese and avocado depending on your desired carb intake.

Grilled Lemon Herb Chicken

Cooking Time: 10-12 minutes |**Prep Time**: 10 minutes |**Total Time**: 20 minutes |**Serving Size**: 4 servings

Ingredients:

- 4 boneless, skinless chicken breasts
- 2 tablespoons olive oil
- 2 lemons, zested and juiced
- 2 cloves garlic, minced
- 1 teaspoon dried thyme
- 1/2 teaspoon dried rosemary
- Salt and pepper to taste

Directions:

1. In a large bowl, whisk together olive oil, lemon zest, lemon juice, garlic, thyme, rosemary, salt, and pepper.
2. Add the chicken breasts to the marinade and toss to coat evenly. Cover and refrigerate for at least 30 minutes, or up to 4 hours.
3. Preheat your grill to medium-high heat.
4. Remove the chicken from the marinade and discard any excess.
5. Grill the chicken for 5-6 minutes per side, or until cooked through and internal temperature reaches 165°F.
6. Serve immediately with your favorite low-carb sides, such as grilled vegetables, roasted cauliflower, or a simple salad.

Nutritional Information per serving: Calories: 250, Fat: 15g, Protein: 30, Carbohydrates: 2g, Fiber: 1g

Tips:

- For added flavor, you can stuff the chicken breasts with fresh herbs like parsley, basil, or oregano before grilling.
- If you don't have a grill, you can bake the chicken in the oven at 400°F for 20-25 minutes, or until cooked through.
- This recipe is also delicious with other types of poultry, such as chicken thighs or turkey breasts.
- For a spicier kick, add a pinch of red pepper flakes to the marinade.

Zucchini Noodles with Pesto and Cherry Tomatoes

Cooking Time: 10 minutes |**Prep Time**: 15 minutes |**Total Time**: 25 minutes |**Serving Size**: 2

Ingredients:

- 2 medium zucchinis
- 1/2 cup fresh basil leaves
- 1/4 cup pine nuts
- 2 cloves garlic
- 1/4 cup olive oil
- 1/4 cup grated Parmesan cheese
- 1/2 teaspoon salt
- 1/4 teaspoon black pepper
- 1 pint cherry tomatoes
- Fresh basil leaves, for garnish (optional)

Directions:

1. Prep the zucchini: Wash and dry the zucchinis. Using a spiralizer, julienne attachment, or vegetable peeler, create long, thin noodles. Set aside.
2. Make the pesto: In a food processor, combine the basil, pine nuts, garlic, olive oil, Parmesan cheese, salt, and pepper. Pulse until a chunky paste forms, scraping down the sides as needed.
3. Cook the zucchini noodles: Heat a large skillet over medium heat. Add the zucchini noodles and cook for 2-3 minutes, stirring occasionally, until slightly softened but still crisp-tender. Do not overcook.
4. Assemble and serve: Transfer the cooked zucchini noodles to a bowl. Add the pesto and toss to coat evenly. Stir in the cherry tomatoes. Garnish with fresh basil leaves, if desired.

Nutritional Information per serving: Calories: 240, Carbohydrates: 8g (net), Fat: 15g, Protein: 8g, Fiber: 3g

Tips:

- For a richer flavor, toast the pine nuts in a dry skillet over medium heat until golden brown, about 3-4 minutes, before adding them to the pesto.
- If you don't have a food processor, you can chop the basil, pine nuts, and garlic finely by hand.
- To make this dish vegan, use a vegan pesto and omit the Parmesan cheese.
- You can add other vegetables to this dish, such as chopped bell peppers, mushrooms, or spinach.
- Leftovers can be stored in an airtight container in the refrigerator for up to 2 days.

Salmon with Avocado Salsa

Cooking time: 10-12 minutes |**Prep time**: 10 minutes |**Total time**: 20 minutes |**Serving size**: 1

Ingredients:

- 1 salmon fillet (6 oz)
- 1/2 avocado, diced
- 1/4 cup cherry tomatoes, diced
- 1/4 red onion, finely chopped
- 1/4 cup cilantro, chopped
- 1 lime, juiced
- 1 tablespoon olive oil
- 1/2 teaspoon chili powder
- 1/4 teaspoon cumin
- 1/4 teaspoon paprika
- Salt and pepper to taste

Directions:

1. Preheat oven to 400°F (200°C). Line a baking sheet with parchment paper.
2. In a small bowl, whisk together olive oil, chili powder, cumin, paprika, salt, and pepper. Rub the mixture onto the salmon fillet.
3. Place the salmon on the prepared baking sheet and bake for 10-12 minutes, or until cooked through.
4. While the salmon is baking, prepare the salsa. In a bowl, combine avocado, tomatoes, red onion, cilantro, and lime juice. Stir gently to combine.
5. To serve, top the cooked salmon with avocado salsa.

Nutritional information per serving: Calories: 450, Fat: 30g, Protein: 40g, Carbohydrates: 5g (3g net carbs)

Tips:

- You can also grill or pan-fry the salmon instead of baking it.
- If you like your salsa spicy, add a jalapeno pepper to the ingredients.
- Serve the salmon with a side of low-carb vegetables, such as roasted Brussels sprouts or asparagus.

Cauliflower Fried Rice

Prep Time: 10 minutes |**Cooking Time**: 15 minutes |**Total Time**: 25 minutes |**Servings**: 2

Ingredients:

- 1 head cauliflower, riced (or 4 cups frozen cauliflower rice)
- 2 tablespoons avocado oil or olive oil
- 2 cloves garlic, minced
- 1 small onion, diced
- 1/2 cup chopped carrots
- 1/2 cup chopped bell pepper
- 1/2 cup frozen peas
- 2 eggs, beaten
- 2 tablespoons soy sauce (or tamari)
- 1 tablespoon rice vinegar
- 1 teaspoon sesame oil
- Salt and pepper to taste
- Green onions, chopped, for garnish (optional)

Directions:

1. Heat the oil in a large skillet or wok over medium-high heat. Add the garlic and onion, and cook until softened, about 3 minutes.
2. Add the carrots and bell pepper, and cook for an additional 2-3 minutes.
3. Add the cauliflower rice and peas, and cook for 5-7 minutes, or until the cauliflower is tender-crisp.
4. Push the cauliflower rice to the sides of the pan and create a well in the center. Pour in the beaten eggs and scramble until cooked through.
5. Stir in the soy sauce, rice vinegar, and sesame oil. Season with salt and pepper to taste.
6. Garnish with chopped green onions, if desired.

Nutritional Information per serving: Calories: 25, Carbs: 5g (net), Fat: 15g, Protein: 15g

Tips:

- For a richer flavor, use chicken broth or bone broth instead of water.
- You can add other vegetables to your liking, such as broccoli, zucchini, or mushrooms.
- If you don't have fresh cauliflower, you can use frozen cauliflower rice. Just be sure to thaw it completely before using.
- Leftovers can be stored in an airtight container in the refrigerator for up to 3 days.

Stuffed Bell Peppers

Cooking time: 30 minute |**Prep time**: 15 minutes |**Total time**: 45 minutes |**Serving size**: 4 peppers

Ingredients:

- 4 bell peppers (any color)
- 1 tablespoon olive oil
- 1 small onion, chopped
- 1 pound ground turkey
- 2 cloves garlic, minced
- 1 teaspoon dried oregano
- 1/2 teaspoon salt
- 1/4 teaspoon black pepper
- 1 cup cauliflower rice
- 1/2 cup shredded cheddar cheese
- 1/4 cup chopped fresh parsley (optional)

Directions:

1. Preheat oven to 375°F (190°C).
2. Cut the tops off the bell peppers and remove the seeds and membranes. Rinse the peppers and set them aside.
3. Heat olive oil in a large skillet over medium heat. Add the onion and cook until softened, about 5 minutes.
4. Add the ground turkey and cook until browned, breaking it up with a spoon. Drain any excess fat.
5. Add the garlic, oregano, salt, and pepper to the skillet and cook for 1 minute.
6. Stir in the cauliflower rice and cook until heated through, about 5 minutes.
7. Remove from heat and stir in the cheese and parsley (if using).
8. Spoon the filling into the bell peppers, packing it in tightly.
9. Place the stuffed peppers in a baking dish and bake for 30 minutes, or until the peppers are tender and the filling is bubbly.

Nutritional information per serving: Calories: 350, Fat: 20g, Carbohydrates: 5g (net), Protein: 30g, Fiber: 3g

Tips:

- You can use any type of ground meat you like, such as beef, chicken, or pork.
- If you don't have cauliflower rice, you can use regular rice or quinoa.
- For a spicier flavor, add a pinch of red pepper flakes to the filling.
- Serve the stuffed peppers with a side of low-carb marinara sauce or ranch dressing.

Eggplant Lasagna

Prep Time: 20 minute |**Cooking Time**: 40 minutes |**Total Time**: 60 minutes |**Serving Size**: 6-8 servings

Ingredients:

- 2 large eggplants (around 1.5 lbs)
- 1 tablespoon olive oil
- Salt and pepper to taste
- 1 pound ground beef or Italian sausage (optional)
- 1 medium onion, chopped
- 2 cloves garlic, minced
- 1 (28-ounce) can crushed tomatoes
- 1 (15-ounce) can diced tomatoes, undrained
- 1 tablespoon dried oregano
- 1 teaspoon dried basil
- 1/2 teaspoon red pepper flakes (optional)
- 15 ounces part-skim ricotta cheese
- 1/2 cup grated Parmesan cheese
- 1 large egg
- 1 cup shredded mozzarella cheese
- Fresh basil, for garnish (optional)

Directions:

1. Preheat oven to 400°F (200°C). Line a baking sheet with parchment paper.
2. Slice eggplants lengthwise into 1/4-inch thick slices. Brush both sides with olive oil and season with salt and pepper. Arrange on the prepared baking sheet and roast for 20 minutes, flipping halfway through.
3. While the eggplant roasts, prepare the sauce. In a large skillet, heat remaining olive oil over medium heat. Add ground beef or sausage and cook until browned, breaking up the meat with a spoon. Drain excess fat.
4. Add onion and garlic to the skillet and cook until softened, about 5 minutes. Stir in crushed tomatoes, diced tomatoes, oregano, basil, and red pepper flakes (if using). Bring to a simmer and cook for 15 minutes, stirring occasionally.
5. In a medium bowl, combine ricotta cheese, Parmesan cheese, and egg. Mix well until smooth.
6. To assemble the lasagna, spread a thin layer of sauce on the bottom of a 9x13 inch baking dish. Top with a layer of roasted eggplant slices, then spread with half of the ricotta mixture. Repeat with another layer of eggplant, sauce, and remaining ricotta mixture.
7. Top with shredded mozzarella cheese and bake for 20-25 minutes, or until the cheese is melted and bubbly. Let cool slightly before serving, garnish with fresh basil (optional).

Nutritional Information per serving: Calories: 350, Fat: 20g, Carbohydrates: 5g (net carbs), Protein: 30g, Fiber: 2g

Tips:

- For a vegetarian version, skip the ground beef or sausage and add chopped mushrooms or bell peppers to the sauce.
- If your eggplant releases a lot of liquid while roasting, drain it off before assembling the lasagna.
- You can use almond flour or crushed pork rinds instead of breadcrumbs for a keto-friendly option.
- Leftovers can be stored in an airtight container in the refrigerator for up to 3 day

Shrimp Stir-Fry

Cooking Time: 10-15 minutes |**Prep Time**: 10 minutes |**Total Time**: 20-25 minutes |**Serving Size**: 2-3

Ingredients:

- 1 tablespoon avocado oil
- 1 pound shrimp, peeled and deveined
- 1/2 teaspoon salt
- 1/4 teaspoon black pepper
- 1 tablespoon sesame oil
- 1 red bell pepper, sliced
- 1 cup broccoli florets
- 1/2 cup snow peas
- 2 cloves garlic, minced
- 1 tablespoon grated ginger
- 1/4 cup coconut aminos (low-carb soy sauce substitute)
- 2 tablespoons rice vinegar
- 1 tablespoon sesame seeds
- 1 tablespoon chopped green onions

Directions:

1. Heat avocado oil in a large skillet or wok over medium-high heat. Add shrimp and cook for 3-5 minutes, or until pink and cooked through. Remove from pan and set aside.
2. Heat sesame oil in the same pan. Add bell pepper, broccoli, and snow peas, and cook for 5-7 minutes, or until slightly tender-crisp.
3. Add garlic and ginger, and cook for 30 seconds until fragrant.
4. Stir in coconut aminos, rice vinegar, and salt and pepper. Bring to a simmer and cook for 1 minute.
5. Return shrimp to the pan and toss to combine. Garnish with sesame seeds and green onions.

Nutritional Information per serving: Calories: 350, Fat: 15g, Carbs: 5g (net), Protein: 30g

Tips:

- You can use any type of shrimp you like for this recipe.
- Feel free to add other low-carb vegetables to the stir-fry, such as zucchini, mushrooms, or onions.
- If you don't have coconut aminos, you can use low-sodium soy sauce.
- Serve this stir-fry over cauliflower rice, zoodles, or quinoa for a complete meal.

Cabbage Rolls

Prep Time: 20 minutes |**Cooking Time**: 1 hour |**Total Time**: 1 hour 20 minutes |**Servings**: 6

Ingredients:
- 1 large head of green cabbage
- 1 tablespoon olive oil
- 1 pound ground beef or turkey
- 1/2 onion, diced
- 2 cloves garlic, minced
- 1 cup cauliflower rice
- 1/2 cup chopped mushrooms (optional)
- 1/4 cup chopped fresh parsley
- 1 teaspoon dried oregano
- 1/2 teaspoon salt
- 1/4 teaspoon black pepper
- 1 (28-ounce) can crushed tomatoes, undrained

Directions:

1. Prep the cabbage: Bring a large pot of salted water to a boil. Carefully remove the core of the cabbage with a sharp knife, leaving the leaves intact. Place the cabbage head in the boiling water for 5 minutes, then remove and let cool slightly. Gently peel off the softened leaves, one at a time. Discard the tough center vein from each leaf.
2. Make the filling: Heat olive oil in a large skillet over medium heat. Add the ground meat and cook until browned, breaking it up with a spoon. Drain any excess fat. Add the onion, garlic, cauliflower rice, and mushrooms (if using). Cook until the onion is softened and the cauliflower rice is heated through, about 5 minutes. Stir in the parsley, oregano, salt, and pepper.
3. Assemble the rolls: Place a spoonful of the filling near the base of each cabbage leaf. Fold the sides of the leaf over the filling, then roll up tightly, tucking in the ends.
4. Bake the rolls: Preheat oven to 375°F (190°C). Pour the crushed tomatoes into a baking dish. Arrange the cabbage rolls, seam-side down, in the dish. Cover the dish with foil and bake for 1 hour, or until the cabbage is tender and the filling is cooked through.
5. Serve and enjoy! Let the cabbage rolls cool slightly before serving. Garnish with additional parsley, if desired.

Nutritional Information per Serving: Calories: 350, Fat: 20g, Protein: 30g, Carbs: 5g (net), Fiber: 3g

Tips:

- For a richer flavor, add 1/4 cup of grated Parmesan cheese to the filling.
- Leftover cabbage rolls can be stored in an airtight container in the refrigerator for up to 3 days. Reheat gently in the oven or microwave.
- This recipe can also be made in a slow cooker. Combine the filling ingredients and cabbage rolls in the slow cooker. Pour the crushed tomatoes over the rolls and cook on low for 6-8 hours.

Cauliflower Crust Pizza

Cooking time: 25-30 minutes |**Prep time**: 15 minutes |**Total time**: 40-45 minutes |**Serving size**: 1

Ingredients:
- Cauliflower crust:
- 2 cups riced cauliflower (fresh or frozen)
- 1/2 cup grated Parmesan cheese
- 1/4 cup almond flour
- 1 large egg, beaten
- 1 teaspoon Italian seasoning
- 1/2 teaspoon garlic powder
- 1/4 teaspoon salt
- 1/4 teaspoon black pepper
- Toppings:
- 1/4 cup low-sugar pizza sauce
- 1 cup shredded mozzarella cheese
- 1/2 cup chopped vegetables of your choice (e.g., bell peppers, mushrooms, onions)
- Fresh herbs (optional)

Directions:
1. Prepare the cauliflower crust:
   If using fresh cauliflower, grate it using a food processor or box grater. If using frozen, thaw completely and squeeze out any excess moisture.
   Microwave the cauliflower in a large bowl for 5 minutes on high power. Drain any excess liquid and let the cauliflower cool slightly.
   Preheat oven to 400°F (200°C).
   In a large bowl, combine the cooked cauliflower, Parmesan cheese, almond flour, egg, Italian seasoning, garlic powder, salt, and pepper. Mix well until a thick dough forms.
   Line a baking sheet with parchment paper and spread the cauliflower dough into a 12-inch circle. Press down firmly to form a compact crust.
   Bake for 20-25 minutes, or until the crust is golden brown and slightly firm.
2. Assemble the pizza:
   Spread the pizza sauce over the pre-baked crust.
   Top with your desired vegetables and sprinkle with mozzarella cheese.
   Bake for an additional 10-15 minutes, or until the cheese is melted and bubbly.
   Garnish with fresh herbs (optional) and serve immediately.

Tips:
- For a crispier crust, preheat your baking sheet before adding the dough.
- If you find the dough is too wet, add more almond flour, 1 tablespoon at a time, until it comes together.
- Feel free to get creative with your toppings! Use any low-carb vegetables and meats you like.
- Leftovers can be stored in the refrigerator for up to 3 days.

Grilled Steak with Chimichurri Sauce

Prep Time: 15 minutes | **Cook Time**: 10-15 minutes | **Total Time**: 25-30 minutes | **Servings**: 2

Ingredients:

- 2 bone-in ribeye steaks (about 1 inch thick)
- 1/2 cup fresh parsley, chopped
- 1/4 cup fresh cilantro, chopped
- 2 cloves garlic, minced
- 1/4 cup olive oil
- 2 tablespoons red wine vinegar
- 1 tablespoon lemon juice
- 1/2 teaspoon dried oregano
- 1/4 teaspoon salt
- 1/4 teaspoon black pepper
- Pinch of red pepper flakes (optional)

Directions:

1. Prepare the chimichurri: In a small bowl, combine the parsley, cilantro, garlic, olive oil, red wine vinegar, lemon juice, oregano, salt, pepper, and red pepper flakes (if using). Stir well to combine. Set aside.
2. Preheat your grill to medium-high heat. If using a charcoal grill, wait until the coals are hot and ashy.
3. Pat the steaks dry with paper towels. Season both sides generously with salt and pepper.
4. Place the steaks on the grill and cook for 4-5 minutes per side for medium-rare, or longer for desired doneness. Be sure to monitor the steaks closely to avoid burning.
5. Remove the steaks from the grill and let them rest for 5-10 minutes before slicing. This allows the juices to redistribute throughout the meat.
6. Slice the steaks against the grain and serve with a generous dollop of chimichurri sauce.

Nutritional Information per serving: Calories: 450, Fat: 30g, Protein: 50g, Carbohydrates: 5g (3g net carbs)

Tips:

- For a thicker chimichurri sauce, pulse the ingredients in a food processor until finely chopped.
- You can substitute flank steak, skirt steak, or hanger steak for the ribeye steaks.
- Serve the grilled steak with a side of low-carb vegetables, such as roasted broccoli, grilled asparagus, or a green salad.
- Leftover chimichurri sauce can be stored in the refrigerator for up to 5 days.

SIDE DISHES

Zucchini Noodles with Pesto

Cook Time: 5 minutes | **Prep Time**: 15 minutes | **Total Time**: 20 minutes | **Serving Size**: 2

Ingredients:

- 2 medium zucchini (approximately 8oz)
- 1/4 cup basil pesto (store-bought or homemade)
- 1/2 cup cherry tomatoes, halved
- 1/4 cup crumbled feta cheese
- 1/4 cup chopped fresh basil
- Pinch of red pepper flakes (optional)
- Extra virgin olive oil
- Salt and freshly ground black pepper to taste

Directions:

1. Spiralize the zucchini: Using a spiralizer, create "noodles" from the zucchini. If you don't have a spiralizer, you can use a julienne peeler or mandoline to create thin strips.
2. Cook the zoodles (optional): This step is optional, but can help soften the zoodles and remove excess moisture. Heat a large skillet over medium heat with a drizzle of olive oil. Add the zoodles and cook for 2-3 minutes, stirring occasionally, until just heated through. Drain any excess liquid from the zoodles.
3. Assemble the dish: In a large bowl, combine the cooked zoodles, pesto, cherry tomatoes, feta cheese, and chopped basil. Toss gently to coat the zoodles with the pesto.
4. Season and serve: Drizzle with a little extra olive oil, season with salt and pepper to taste, and garnish with a pinch of red pepper flakes (optional). Serve immediately.

Nutritional Information per serving: Calories: 200, Carbs: 8g (net), Fat: 15g, Protein: 4g

Tips:

- If you're short on time, use store-bought pesto. However, for extra flavor, consider making your own.
- For additional protein, add grilled chicken, shrimp, or tofu.
- This dish can be served hot or cold. Leftovers can be stored in an airtight container in the refrigerator for up to 2 days.
- Feel free to get creative with the vegetables! Add other low-carb favorites like shredded bell peppers, roasted asparagus, or sun-dried tomatoes.

Cauliflower "Potato" Salad

Prep Time: 10 minutes | **Cook Time**: 15 minutes | **Total Time**: 25 minutes | **Servings**: 4-6

Ingredients:

- 1 head cauliflower, cut into florets
- 1/2 cup mayonnaise (use avocado mayo for extra creaminess)
- 2 tablespoons Dijon mustard
- 1 tablespoon apple cider vinegar
- 1/2 teaspoon garlic powder
- 1/2 teaspoon paprika
- 1/4 teaspoon salt
- 1/4 teaspoon black pepper
- 1/3 cup red onion, finely diced
- 1/3 cup celery, thinly sliced
- 2 hard-boiled eggs, chopped
- Chives, for garnish (optional)

Directions:

1. Choose your cooking method: You can either roast the cauliflower for a richer flavor (15 minutes at 400°F) or steam it for a lighter option (10 minutes).

2. Prepare the cauliflower: While the cauliflower cooks, whisk together the mayonnaise, Dijon mustard, apple cider vinegar, garlic powder, paprika, salt, and pepper in a bowl.

3. Cool and chop: Once cooked, let the cauliflower cool slightly, then chop it into bite-sized pieces.

4. Assemble the salad: In a large bowl, combine the cooled cauliflower, mayonnaise dressing, red onion, celery, and hard-boiled eggs. Toss gently to coat.

5. Chill and garnish: Refrigerate the salad for at least 30 minutes to allow the flavors to meld. Garnish with chives before serving, if desired.

Nutritional Information per serving: Calories: 150, Fat: 12g, Carbohydrates: 4g (net), Fiber: 3g, Protein: 5g

Tips:

- For a tangy flavor, add a tablespoon of dill pickles or relish to the dressing.
- If you like it spicy, add a pinch of cayenne pepper to the dressing.
- Feel free to customize the vegetables! Add in chopped bell peppers, cucumbers, or radishes for additional flavor and crunch.
- Leftovers can be stored in an airtight container in the refrigerator for up to 3 days.

Asparagus Wrapped in Prosciutto

Prep Time: 10 minutes | **Cook Time**: 10 minutes | **Total Time**: 20 minutes | **Servings**: 4

Ingredients:

- 1 pound asparagus spears, trimmed
- 8 slices prosciutto, thinly sliced
- 1 tablespoon olive oil
- Freshly ground black pepper, to taste

Directions:

1. Preheat oven to 400°F (200°C). Line a baking sheet with parchment paper.

2. Trim the asparagus spears by snapping off the woody ends.

3. Drizzle the asparagus with olive oil and season with black pepper.

4. Lay a prosciutto slice flat on a cutting board. Place an asparagus spear at the bottom of the prosciutto slice and roll up, starting from the bottom and continuing to the tip.

5. Repeat with remaining asparagus spears and prosciutto slices.

6. Arrange the wrapped asparagus on the prepared baking sheet.

7. Bake for 10-12 minutes, or until the prosciutto is crisp and the asparagus is tender-crisp.

8. Serve immediately.

Nutritional Information per serving: Calories: 70, Fat: 5g, Carbohydrates: 3g (1g net carbs), Protein: 6g, Fiber: 2g

Tips:

- For a vegetarian option, you can use thinly sliced zucchini or eggplant instead of prosciutto.
- You can also grill the asparagus wrapped in prosciutto for a smoky flavor.
- To add a bit of sweetness, you can drizzle the asparagus with balsamic glaze before serving.

Stuffed Mushrooms

Prep Time: 15 minutes | **Cooking Time**: 20-25 minutes | **Total Time**: 40-45 minutes | **Serving Size**: 12-14 mushrooms

Ingredients:

- 12-14 large portobello mushrooms or cremini mushrooms
- 2 tablespoons olive oil
- 1/2 onion, finely chopped
- 2 cloves garlic, minced
- 1/2 pound ground sausage or ground turkey (optional)
- 4 ounces cream cheese, softened
- 1/2 cup shredded parmesan cheese
- 1/4 cup chopped fresh herbs (parsley, basil, oregano, thyme)
- Salt and pepper to taste

Directions:

1. Preheat oven to 375°F (190°C). Line a baking sheet with parchment paper.
2. Gently remove the stems from the mushrooms and finely chop them.
3. In a large skillet, heat olive oil over medium heat. Add the onion and cook until softened, about 5 minutes.
4. Add the garlic and cook for 1 minute more until fragrant.
5. If using, add the ground sausage or turkey and cook until browned. Drain any excess fat.
6. Stir in the chopped mushroom stems and cook until softened, about 5 minutes.
7. Remove from heat and let cool slightly.
8. In a bowl, combine the softened cream cheese, parmesan cheese, herbs, salt, and pepper.
9. Add the cooled mushroom mixture and stir to combine.
10. Spoon the filling into the mushroom caps, packing it in gently.
11. Place the stuffed mushrooms on the prepared baking sheet.
12. Bake for 20-25 minutes, or until the mushrooms are tender and the filling is bubbly and golden brown.
13. Serve immediately, garnished with additional herbs if desired.

Nutritional Information per Serving: Calories: 150-200, Fat: 10-15g, Protein: 10-15g, Carbohydrates: 5-10g (net carbs)

Tips:

- For a vegetarian option, omit the sausage or turkey and add additional chopped vegetables to the filling, such as bell peppers, zucchini, or spinach.
- If you don't have cream cheese, you can use ricotta cheese or mascarpone cheese as a substitute.
- You can also grill the stuffed mushrooms for a smoky flavor. Preheat your grill to medium-high heat and cook the mushrooms for 10-15 minutes per side, or until tender.
- To make this dish ahead of time, prepare the filling and stuff the mushrooms. Cover and refrigerate for up to 24 hours. Bake as directed before serving.

Cucumber Avocado Salad

Cooking Time: None | **Prep Time**: 10 minutes | **Total Time**: 10 minutes | **Serving Size**: 4

Nutritional Information per Serving: Calories: 230, Fat: 18g (13g saturated), Carbohydrates: 5g (2g fiber), Protein: 2g, Sodium: 130mg

Ingredients:

- 1 English cucumber, thinly sliced
- 1 ripe avocado, diced
- 1/2 red onion, finely diced (optional)
- 1/4 cup chopped fresh cilantro
- 2 tablespoons olive oil
- 2 tablespoons lime juice
- Salt and pepper to taste

Optional additions:
- Chopped cherry tomatoes
- Crumbled feta cheese
- Sliced jalapeño peppers
- Fresh herbs like basil or mint

Directions:

1. Prep the vegetables: Thinly slice the English cucumber and dice the avocado. If using red onion, finely chop it.

2. Combine the ingredients: In a large bowl, combine the cucumber, avocado, red onion (if using), and cilantro.

3. Make the dressing: In a small bowl, whisk together the olive oil, lime juice, salt, and pepper.

4. Dress the salad: Pour the dressing over the salad and toss gently to coat.

5. Serve immediately: Enjoy the salad as is, or top with your favorite optional ingredients.

Tips:

- To prevent the avocado from browning, toss it with a little lime juice before adding it to the salad.
- If you don't have English cucumber, you can use regular cucumber, but be sure to remove the seeds first as they can be bitter.
- This salad is best enjoyed fresh, but you can store it in the refrigerator for up to a day. Just be aware that the avocado may brown a little.

Grilled Eggplant with Feta

Cooking Time: 10-12 minutes | **Prep Time**: 10 minutes | **Total Time**: 20-22 minutes | **Serving Size**: 2

Ingredients:

- 1 medium eggplant (about 1 pound)
- 2 tablespoons olive oil
- 1/2 teaspoon dried oregano
- 1/4 teaspoon red pepper flakes (optional)
- Salt and freshly ground black pepper to taste
- 4 ounces feta cheese, crumbled
- 1/4 cup chopped fresh parsley (optional)
- 1 tablespoon lemon juice (optional)

Directions:

1. Prepare the eggplant: Wash the eggplant and cut it into 1/2-inch thick slices. If desired, sprinkle the slices with salt and let them sit for 15-20 minutes to draw out any bitterness. Rinse and pat dry with paper towels.
2. Marinate the eggplant: In a large bowl, combine olive oil, oregano, red pepper flakes (if using), salt, and pepper. Add the eggplant slices and toss to coat evenly.
3. Grill the eggplant: Preheat your grill to medium-high heat. Lightly oil the grates if needed. Place the eggplant slices on the grill and cook for 3-4 minutes per side, or until tender and slightly charred.
4. Assemble and serve: Transfer the grilled eggplant to a serving platter. Top with crumbled feta cheese, chopped parsley (if using), and a drizzle of lemon juice (if using). Serve immediately while warm.

Nutritional Information per serving: Calories: 160, Fat: 13g (9g saturated), Carbs: 6g (3g net carbs), Fiber: 3g, Protein: 7g

Tips:

- For a thicker sauce, you can mash some of the feta cheese with a fork and spread it over the eggplant before adding the crumbled cheese.
- You can grill zucchini or other vegetables alongside the eggplant for a more colorful and varied side dish.
- This dish can be made ahead of time and served at room temperature.
- To make this dish vegan, simply omit the feta cheese and drizzle with a balsamic reduction or tahini sauce.

Broccoli Salad with Bacon and Cheddar

Cooking time: 10 minutes | **Prep time**: 15 minutes | **Total time**: 25 minutes | **Serving size**: 4-6 servings

Ingredients:

- 1 head of broccoli, cut into florets
- 4 slices of bacon, cooked and crumbled
- 1/2 cup shredded cheddar cheese
- 1/4 cup red onion, thinly sliced
- 2 tablespoons mayonnaise
- 1 tablespoon apple cider vinegar
- 1/2 teaspoon Dijon mustard
- Salt and pepper to taste

Directions:

1. In a large bowl, combine the broccoli, bacon, cheddar cheese, and red onion.

2. In a small bowl, whisk together the mayonnaise, apple cider vinegar, Dijon mustard, salt, and pepper.

3. Pour the dressing over the broccoli mixture and toss to coat.

4. Serve immediately.

Nutritional information per serving: Calories: 300, Fat: 22g, Carbohydrates: 5g (3g net carbs), Protein: 20g

Tips:

- For a more flavorful salad, roast the broccoli florets in the oven for 10-15 minutes before adding them to the salad.
- You can also add other chopped vegetables to the salad, such as celery, carrots, or bell peppers.
- If you don't have Dijon mustard, you can substitute with regular mustard.
- This salad can be stored in the refrigerator for up to 3 days.

Cauliflower Rice Stir-Fry

Prep Time: 10 minutes | **Cook Time**: 15 minutes | **Total Time**: 25 minutes | **Servings**: 4

Ingredients:

- 1 head cauliflower, riced
- 1 tablespoon avocado oil
- 1/2 cup chopped onion
- 2 cloves garlic, minced
- 1 red bell pepper, sliced
- 1 cup broccoli florets
- 1/2 cup chopped mushrooms
- 1/4 cup chopped green onions
- 2 tablespoons low-sodium soy sauce
- 1 tablespoon rice vinegar
- 1 teaspoon sesame oil
- 1/2 teaspoon sriracha (optional)
- Salt and pepper to taste

Directions:

1. Prep the cauliflower rice: If using fresh cauliflower, wash and grate it using the large holes of a box grater. Alternatively, pulse the cauliflower florets in a food processor until rice-sized. If using frozen cauliflower rice, thaw it according to package instructions.
2. Heat the oil in a large skillet or wok over medium-high heat. Add the onion and cook until softened, about 5 minutes.
3. Add the garlic and cook for 30 seconds until fragrant.
4. Stir in the bell pepper, broccoli, and mushrooms. Cook for 5-7 minutes, or until the vegetables are slightly tender-crisp.
5. Add the cauliflower rice and cook for 2-3 minutes, stirring constantly, until heated through.
6. In a small bowl, whisk together the soy sauce, rice vinegar, sesame oil, and sriracha (if using). Pour the sauce into the pan and stir to combine.
7. Season with salt and pepper to taste. Garnish with chopped green onions and serve immediately.

Nutritional Information per Serving: Calories: 220, Carbohydrates: 10g (net), Fiber: 4g, Protein: 15g, Fat: 10g

Tips:

- For a protein boost, add cooked chicken, shrimp, or tofu to the stir-fry.
- Feel free to experiment with different vegetables, such as zucchini, carrots, or snap peas.
- If you don't have rice vinegar, you can substitute with white vinegar or lemon juice.
- Leftovers can be stored in an airtight container in the refrigerator for up to 3 days.

Spaghetti Squash with Marinara Sauce

Prep Time: 10 minutes | **Cook Time**: 45 minutes | **Total Time**: 55 minutes | **Servings**: 4

Ingredients:

- 1 medium spaghetti squash
- 1 tablespoon olive oil
- Salt and pepper to taste
- 1 (28-ounce) can crushed tomatoes
- 1 clove garlic, minced
- 1/2 teaspoon dried oregano
- 1/4 teaspoon red pepper flakes (optional)
- 1/4 cup chopped fresh basil (optional)
- Grated Parmesan cheese, for serving

Directions:

1. Preheat oven to 400°F (200°C).
2. Cut the spaghetti squash in half lengthwise and scoop out the seeds. Drizzle the cut sides with olive oil and season with salt and pepper.
3. Place the squash halves cut-side down on a baking sheet and roast for 40-45 minutes, or until tender.
4. While the squash is roasting, make the marinara sauce. In a saucepan, heat the olive oil over medium heat. Add the garlic and cook for 30 seconds, until fragrant.
5. Stir in the crushed tomatoes, oregano, and red pepper flakes (if using). Bring to a simmer and cook for 15 minutes, stirring occasionally.
6. Once the squash is done, remove from the oven and let cool slightly. Use a fork to scrape out the spaghetti-like strands.
7. Divide the spaghetti squash among plates and top with the marinara sauce. Garnish with fresh basil and Parmesan cheese, if desired.

Nutritional Information per serving: Calories: 280, Carbohydrates: 12g (net), Fiber: 5g, Protein: 10g, Fat: 10g

Tips:

- For a richer flavor, use fire-roasted crushed tomatoes.
- You can also add other vegetables to the marinara sauce, such as chopped onions, peppers, or mushrooms.
- If you don't have fresh basil, you can use 1 teaspoon dried basil.
- Leftovers can be stored in an airtight container in the refrigerator for up to 3 days.

Brussels sprouts with Bacon and Almonds

Cooking Time: 20 minutes | **Prep Time**: 10 minutes | **Total Time**: 30 minutes | **Serving Size**: 4-6 servings

Ingredients:

- 1 pound Brussels sprouts, trimmed and halved
- 4 slices bacon, chopped
- 1/4 cup sliced almonds
- 2 tablespoons olive oil
- 1/2 teaspoon dried thyme
- 1/4 teaspoon red pepper flakes (optional)
- Salt and pepper to taste

Directions:

1. Preheat oven to 400°F (200°C).
2. In a large bowl, toss the Brussels sprouts with olive oil, thyme, red pepper flakes (if using), salt, and pepper.
3. Spread the Brussels sprouts on a baking sheet in a single layer.
4. Roast for 15-20 minutes, or until tender and slightly browned.
5. Meanwhile, cook the bacon in a skillet over medium heat until crispy. Drain on paper towels, then crumble.
6. Toast the almonds in the same skillet over medium heat until golden brown, about 3-4 minutes.
7. Once the Brussels sprouts are roasted, add the bacon and almonds to the baking sheet and toss to combine.
8. Serve immediately and enjoy!

Nutritional Information per serving: Calories: 180, Fat: 13g, Carbohydrates: 5g (2g net carbs), Protein: 12g, Fiber: 3g

Tips:

- For a sweeter flavor, add a drizzle of balsamic glaze or a sprinkle of dried cranberries before serving.
- If you don't have bacon, you can substitute pancetta or chorizo for a similar flavor.
- You can also add other vegetables to this dish, such as chopped broccoli, cauliflower, or bell peppers.
- To make this dish ahead of time, roast the Brussels sprouts and then store them in an airtight container in the refrigerator for up to 3 days. Reheat them in the oven before serving.

Chocolate Avocado Mousse

Prep Time: 10 minutes | **Cooking Time**: None | **Total Time**: 10 minutes | **Serving Size**: 4

Ingredients:

- 2 ripe avocados
- 1/4 cup unsweetened cocoa powder
- 2 tablespoons sweetener of choice (monk fruit sweetener, erythritol, stevia)
- 1/4 cup unsweetened almond milk
- 1 teaspoon vanilla extract
- Pinch of sea salt

Optional Toppings:
- Whipped cream (keto-friendly)
- Chopped nuts
- Berries
- Shredded coconut

Directions:

1. Scoop and Blend: Halve and pit the avocados, scooping out the flesh into a blender. Add the cocoa powder, sweetener, almond milk, vanilla extract, and sea salt. Blend until smooth and creamy, scraping down the sides as needed.

2. Chill and Serve: Divide the mousse evenly among 4 ramekins or small bowls. Cover and refrigerate for at least 2 hours, or until set. Top with your favorite garnishes and enjoy!

Nutritional Information per Serving: Calories: 220, Fat: 18g, Carbohydrates: 3g, Protein: 4g, Sugar: 1g

Tips:

- For an extra rich mousse, use full-fat coconut milk instead of almond milk.
- If your mousse is too thick, add a tablespoon or two of milk until it reaches desired consistency.
- Get creative with your toppings! Fresh berries, a drizzle of sugar-free chocolate syrup, or a sprinkle of chopped nuts are all delicious options.

Berry Chia Seed Pudding

Prep Time: 5 minutes | **Cooking Time**: 0 minutes | **Total Time**: 2 hours or more | **Serving Size**: 1

Ingredients:

- 1/4 cup chia seeds
- 1 cup unsweetened almond milk (or another low-carb milk)
- 1/4 cup fresh or frozen berries
- 1/2 teaspoon vanilla extract (optional)
- 1/4 teaspoon stevia or monk fruit sweetener (optional)
- Toppings (optional): additional berries, chopped nuts, shredded coconut, or a dollop of whipped cream

Directions:

1. In a small bowl or jar, whisk together the chia seeds, almond milk, vanilla extract (if using), and sweetener (if using).

2. Add the berries.

3. Cover the bowl or jar and refrigerate for at least 2 hours, or overnight. The chia seeds will absorb the liquid and thicken into a pudding consistency.

4. When ready to serve, stir the pudding and top with your desired toppings.

Nutritional Information per serving: Calories: 230, Fat: 13g, Carbohydrates: 8g (net 3g), Fiber: 5g, Protein: 6g

Tips:

- For a thicker pudding, use less milk. For a thinner pudding, use more milk.
- You can use any type of berries you like.
- If you don't have fresh berries, you can use frozen berries. Just thaw them slightly before adding them to the pudding.
- For extra flavor, you can add a pinch of cinnamon or nutmeg to the pudding.
- This pudding is also great for meal prep. Make a batch ahead of time and store it in the refrigerator for up to 5 days.

Coconut Flour Pancakes

Cooking Time: 10-12 minutes | **Prep Time**: 5 minutes | **Total Time**: 15 minutes | **Serving Size**: 8 pancakes

Ingredients:

- 1/4 cup coconut flour
- 1/2 teaspoon baking powder
- 1/4 teaspoon salt
- 2 large eggs
- 2 tablespoons almond milk (unsweetened)
- 1 tablespoon melted coconut oil
- 1 tablespoon honey or maple syrup (optional)
- 1/2 teaspoon vanilla extract

Directions:

1. In a medium bowl, whisk together the coconut flour, baking powder, and salt.

2. In a separate bowl, whisk together the eggs, almond milk, coconut oil, honey or maple syrup (if using), and vanilla extract.

3. Add the wet ingredients to the dry ingredients and whisk until just combined. Let the batter sit for 5 minutes to thicken.

4. Heat a greased griddle or skillet over medium heat. Pour about 1/4 cup of batter per pancake onto the griddle.

5. Cook for 2-3 minutes per side, or until golden brown.

6. Serve immediately with your favorite toppings, such as fresh fruit, whipped cream, or nut butter.

Nutritional Information per pancake: Calories: 130, Fat: 8g, Carbs: 5g (net), Fiber: 3g, Protein: 7g

Tips:

- For extra fluffiness, separate the eggs and beat the whites until stiff peaks form, then gently fold them into the batter.
- If the batter is too thick, add a little more almond milk. If it's too thin, add a little more coconut flour.
- These pancakes are best served fresh, but they can also be stored in an airtight container in the refrigerator for up to 3 days. Reheat them in a skillet over low heat or in the microwave.

Greek Yogurt with Nuts and Berries

Cooking Time: None | **Prep Time**: 5 minutes | **Total Time**: 5 minutes | **Serving Size**: 1 bowl

Ingredients:

- 1 cup plain Greek yogurt (full-fat or 2% fat)
- 1/2 cup mixed berries (blueberries, raspberries, strawberries)
- 1/4 cup chopped nuts (almonds, pecans, walnuts)
- 1/4 teaspoon vanilla extract (optional)
- Stevia or monk fruit sweetener to taste (optional)
- Fresh mint leaves for garnish (optional)

Directions:

1. Prep the fruit and nuts: If using frozen berries, thaw them slightly. Chop the nuts to your desired size.

2. Assemble the bowl: In a serving bowl, scoop in the Greek yogurt. Top with the berries and nuts, spreading them evenly.

3. Flavor to your liking: Drizzle with vanilla extract if desired. Adjust the sweetness with stevia or monk fruit sweetener to your taste.

4. Garnish and enjoy: Top with fresh mint leaves for a pop of color and freshness. Dig in and savor your guilt-free, low-carb dessert!

Nutritional Information per serving: Calories: 250, Fat: 14g (healthy fats), Carbohydrates: 10g (5g net carbs), Protein: 20g, Fiber: 5g

Tips:

- For extra protein and fiber, sprinkle some chia seeds or ground flaxseed on top.
- Use different types of nuts and berries for variety in flavor and texture.
- If you prefer a warmer treat, heat the berries in a small saucepan with a splash of water or lemon juice before adding them to the yogurt.
- This recipe is easily doubled or tripled to serve a crowd.

Sugar-Free Cheesecake

Prep Time: 15 minutes | **Cook Time**: 50-60 minutes | **Total Time**: 4 hours 15 minutes | **Servings**: 10-12 slices

Ingredients:

Crust:
- 1 1/4 cups almond flour
- 3 tablespoons melted butter
- 1/2 teaspoon ground cinnamon
- Pinch of salt

Filling:
- 24 ounces full-fat cream cheese, softened
- 1/2 cup granulated erythritol or monk fruit sweetener (or to taste)
- 3 large eggs
- 1/3 cup sour cream
- 1 tablespoon lemon juice
- 1 teaspoon vanilla extract

Directions:

1. Preheat oven to 350°F (175°C). Line the bottom of a 9-inch spring form pan with parchment paper.
2. Make the crust: In a medium bowl, combine almond flour, melted butter, cinnamon, and salt. Mix until crumbly and press into the bottom of the prepared pan. Bake for 10-12 minutes, or until lightly golden. Let cool completely.
3. Make the filling: In a large bowl, beat cream cheese and sweetener until light and fluffy. Beat in eggs one at a time, then stir in sour cream, lemon juice, and vanilla extract until smooth.
4. Pour filling over the cooled crust. Bake for 50-60 minutes, or until the edges are set but the center is still slightly jiggly.
5. Turn off the oven and crack open the door slightly. Let the cheesecake cool in the oven for 1 hour, then transfer to the refrigerator and chill for at least 4 hours, or overnight, until set.
6. Serve chilled and enjoy! You can top your cheesecake with fresh berries, whipped cream, or a drizzle of sugar-free chocolate syrup for an extra decadent treat.

Nutritional Information per Serving: Calories: 250, Fat: 20g, Carbohydrates: 4g (net carbs 2g), Protein: 8g

Tips:
- For a richer flavor, use full-fat cream cheese and sour cream.
- If your cheesecake cracks slightly on top, don't worry! It's perfectly normal. You can cover any cracks with whipped cream or fruit topping.
- To ensure the cheesecake sets properly, it's important to let it cool completely in the oven before refrigerating.
- Store leftover cheesecake in the refrigerator for up to 3 days.

Dark Chocolate Bark

Prep Time: 10 minutes | **Cooking Time**: 5 minutes | **Total Time**: 15 minutes | **Servings**: 12-15 pieces

Ingredients:

- 8 ounces sugar-free dark chocolate chips (70% cacao or higher)
- 1 tablespoon coconut oil
- 1/4 cup chopped almonds
- 1/4 cup chopped walnuts
- 1/4 cup chopped pecans
- 1/4 cup unsweetened shredded coconut
- 1/4 cup dried cranberries (optional)
- Sea salt flakes, for garnish

Directions:

1. Prepare the baking sheet. Line a baking sheet with parchment paper.

2. Melt the chocolate. In a heat-proof bowl set over a pan of simmering water (don't let the bowl touch the water), melt the chocolate chips and coconut oil together, stirring occasionally, until smooth.

3. Pour and top. Pour the melted chocolate onto the prepared baking sheet and spread it into an even layer. Sprinkle with the chopped nuts, coconut, cranberries (if using), and a pinch of sea salt.

4. Chill and break. Refrigerate the bark for at least 2 hours, or until firm. Break into pieces and enjoy!

Nutritional Information per serving: Calories: 150, Fat: 12g (7g saturated), Net Carbs: 4g, Fiber: 3g, Protein: 2g

Tips:

- For a richer flavor, use a higher-cocoa percentage chocolate (80% or higher).
- Get creative with the toppings! Try other nuts, seeds, dried fruit, or even crushed mint candies.
- Store leftover bark in an airtight container in the refrigerator for up to a week.

Peanut Butter Protein Balls

Cooking Time: None | **Prep Time**: 10 minutes | **Total Time**: 10 minutes | **Serving Size**: 10-12 balls

Ingredients:

- 1/2 cup unsweetened natural peanut butter
- 1/4 cup unsweetened almond flour
- 1/4 cup coconut flour
- 2 tablespoons protein powder (choose a low-carb brand)
- 1 tablespoon chia seeds
- 1 tablespoon ground flaxseed
- 1 tablespoon honey or maple syrup (optional)
- 1/4 teaspoon sea salt
- 1/2 cup chopped nuts or dark chocolate chips (optional)

Directions:

1. In a large bowl, combine the peanut butter, almond flour, coconut flour, protein powder, chia seeds, flaxseed, honey or maple syrup (if using), and sea salt. Mix well until a thick dough forms.

2. Add the chopped nuts or dark chocolate chips (if using) and stir until evenly distributed.

3. Roll the dough into 10-12 balls.

4. Place the balls on a baking sheet lined with parchment paper and refrigerate for at least 30 minutes, or until firm.

5. Enjoy!

Nutritional Information per serving: Calories: 180, Fat: 10g (healthy fats!), Carbs: 5g (net carbs), Fiber: 3g, Protein: 8g

Tips:

- You can store these balls in an airtight container in the refrigerator for up to a week.
- If the dough is too dry, add a teaspoon of water at a time until it becomes sticky and moldable.
- Feel free to get creative with the add-ins! Other tasty options include dried fruit, shredded coconut, or spices like cinnamon or nutmeg.

Low-Carb Fruit Salad

Cooking Time: None | **Prep Time**: 10 minutes | **Total Time**: 10 minutes | **Serving Size**: 4-6

Ingredients:

- 1 cup sliced strawberries
- 1 cup raspberries
- 1 cup blueberries
- 1/2 cup blackberries
- 1/4 cup cantaloupe cubes
- 1/4 cup honeydew melon cubes
- 1/4 cup chopped kiwi
- 1/4 cup chopped avocado
- 1/4 cup chopped walnuts (optional)
- 2 tablespoons fresh lime juice
- 1 tablespoon stevia powder (or to taste)
- 1/4 teaspoon vanilla extract
- Pinch of fresh mint (optional)

Directions:

1. Wash and chop all fruits. Slice the strawberries, cantaloupe, and honeydew melon. Chop the raspberries, blueberries, blackberries, kiwi, and avocado.
2. Combine fruits in a large bowl. Gently toss together the chopped strawberries, raspberries, blueberries, blackberries, kiwi, cantaloupe, honeydew melon, and avocado.
3. Prepare the dressing. In a small bowl, whisk together the lime juice, stevia powder, vanilla extract, and mint (if using).
4. Drizzle the dressing over the fruit salad. Gently stir to distribute the dressing evenly.
5. Top with walnuts (optional) and serve immediately. Enjoy your refreshing and guilt-free low-carb fruit salad!

Nutritional Information per Serving: Calories: 150, Carbs: 5g (net), Fat: 2g, Protein: 2g, Fiber: 3g

Tips:

- For a creamier texture, you can stir in 1/4 cup of unsweetened plain Greek yogurt.
- Adjust the sweetness of the dressing to your preference. You can use a different low-carb sweetener like erythritol or monk fruit sweetener if desired.
- Substitute or add other low-carb fruits like oranges, grapefruit, starfruit, or diced apples.
- Make it a festive appetizer by skewering the fruit pieces and drizzling with the dressing.
- This salad is best enjoyed fresh, but it will keep in the refrigerator for up to 24 hours.

Zucchini Bread

Prep Time: 10 minutes | **Cooking Time**: 50-60 minutes | **Total Time**: 1 hour | **Servings**: 10 slices

Ingredients:

- 1 1/2 cups grated zucchini, squeezed dry
- 1/4 cup melted coconut oil
- 3 large eggs
- 1/2 cup almond flour
- 1/4 cup coconut flour
- 1/4 cup monk fruit sweetener or erythritol
- 1 1/2 teaspoons baking powder
- 1 teaspoon ground cinnamon
- 1/2 teaspoon sea salt
- 1/4 teaspoon nutmeg (optional)
- 1/4 cup chopped walnuts or pecans (optional)

Directions:

1. Preheat oven to 350°F (175°C) and grease a 9x5 inch loaf pan.
2. In a large bowl, whisk together the grated zucchini, melted coconut oil, and eggs.
3. In a separate bowl, whisk together the almond flour, coconut flour, sweetener, baking powder, cinnamon, salt, and nutmeg (if using).
4. Add the dry ingredients to the wet ingredients and stir until just combined. Fold in the chopped nuts, if using.
5. Pour the batter into the prepared loaf pan and smooth the top.
6. Bake for 50-60 minutes, or until a toothpick inserted into the center comes out clean.
7. Let the bread cool in the pan for 10 minutes, then transfer it to a wire rack to cool completely before slicing and serving.

Nutritional Information per slice: Calories: 150, Fat: 10g, Carbohydrates: 5g (net), Fiber: 3g, Protein: 5g

Tips:

- For extra moisture, you can add 1/4 cup of unsweetened applesauce to the batter.
- If you don't have monk fruit sweetener or erythritol, you can use stevia to taste.
- You can also add other mix-ins to the bread, such as chocolate chips, dried fruit, or shredded carrots.
- Store leftovers in an airtight container in the refrigerator for up to 5 days.

Avocado Chocolate Truffles

Cooking Time: 5 minutes | **Prep Time**: 10 minutes | **Total Time**: 15 minutes | **Serving Size**: 12 truffles

Ingredients:

- 1/2 cup mashed ripe avocado (about 1/2 medium avocado)
- 3 oz unsweetened dark chocolate, chopped
- 1 tablespoon coconut oil
- 1/4 teaspoon vanilla extract
- Pinch of sea salt
- Cocoa powder, for dusting (optional)

Directions:

1. Melt the chocolate: Place the chopped chocolate and coconut oil in a heat-safe bowl over a saucepan of simmering water (double boiler). Stir constantly until melted and smooth. Alternatively, microwave in 30-second intervals, stirring in between, until melted.

2. Combine ingredients: In a food processor or blender, combine the melted chocolate mixture, mashed avocado, vanilla extract, and salt. Process until smooth and creamy, scraping down the sides as needed.

3. Chill and form truffles: Transfer the mixture to a bowl and place in the refrigerator for at least 30 minutes, or until firm enough to roll. Using a tablespoon or your hands, roll the mixture into 12 small balls.

4. Dust and enjoy: Place cocoa powder in a shallow dish. Roll each truffle in the cocoa powder to coat, if desired. Enjoy immediately or store in the refrigerator for up to 3 days.

Nutritional Information per truffle: Calories: 130, Fat: 11g (6g saturated), Net Carbs: 2g, Fiber: 2g, Protein: 1g

Tips:

- For a richer truffle flavor, use 70% or higher dark chocolate.
- You can also add a pinch of chili powder or cinnamon to the mixture for a spiced twist.
- If the mixture is too soft to roll after chilling, try placing it in the freezer for 10-15 minutes.
- To make the truffles look extra fancy, dip them in melted dark chocolate before rolling in cocoa powder.

SEAFOOD

Salmon

Cooking Time: 10-12 minutes | **Prep Time**: 5 minutes | **Total Time**: 15 minutes | **Serving Size**: 1 fillet

Ingredients:

- 1 salmon fillet (6-8oz)
- 1 tablespoon olive oil
- 1/2 teaspoon dried oregano
- 1/4 teaspoon garlic powder
- 1/4 teaspoon salt
- 1/4 teaspoon black pepper
- 1/2 lemon, sliced
- 1 bunch asparagus, trimmed
- Optional: fresh parsley, for garnish

Directions:

1. Preheat a large skillet over medium-high heat.
2. Pat the salmon fillet dry with paper towels and season with oregano, garlic powder, salt, and pepper.
3. Heat the olive oil in the skillet until shimmering. Add the salmon fillet, skin-side down, and cook for 3-4 minutes, or until the skin is crispy and golden brown.
4. Flip the salmon and add the lemon slices to the pan. Reduce heat to medium and cook for an additional 3-4 minutes, or until the salmon is cooked through.
5. While the salmon is cooking, roast the asparagus. Toss the asparagus with a drizzle of olive oil, salt, and pepper. Spread on a baking sheet and roast in a preheated oven at 400°F for 10-12 minutes, or until tender-crisp.
6. Plate the salmon and asparagus, drizzle with pan juices, and garnish with fresh parsley (optional).

Nutritional Information per serving: Calories: 420, Fat: 25g, Carbohydrates: 4g (net), Protein: 40g

Tips:

- If you prefer, you can bake the salmon instead of pan-searing it. Preheat the oven to 400°F and bake the salmon for 10-12 minutes, or until cooked through.
- For a richer flavor, you can add a tablespoon of butter to the pan when you cook the salmon.
- Serve this dish with a side of low-carb rice or quinoa, or with a simple salad.

Garlic Lemon Butter Shrimp with Zucchini Noodles

Prep Time: 10 minutes | **Cooking Time**: 15 minutes | **Total Time**: 25 minutes | **Serving Size**: 2

Ingredients:

- 1 pound large shrimp, peeled and deveined
- 1 tablespoon olive oil
- 2 cloves garlic, minced
- 1/2 teaspoon dried oregano
- 1/4 teaspoon salt
- 1/4 teaspoon black pepper
- 1/2 lemon, juiced
- 2 tablespoons butter
- 2 medium zucchini, spiralized into noodles
- Fresh parsley, chopped (optional)

Directions:

1. In a medium bowl, toss the shrimp with olive oil, garlic, oregano, salt, pepper, and lemon juice. Marinate for at least 10 minutes.

2. While the shrimp marinates, heat a large skillet over medium-high heat. Melt the butter.

3. Add the zucchini noodles and cook for 5-7 minutes, stirring occasionally, until tender-crisp.

4. Add the marinated shrimp to the skillet and cook for 3-4 minutes per side, or until pink and opaque.

5. Remove the pan from heat and garnish with fresh parsley, if desired.

6. Serve immediately and enjoy!

Nutritional Information per serving: Calories: 300, Fat: 14g (2g saturated), Protein: 30g, Carbohydrates: 5g (3g net carbs), Fiber: 2g

Tips:

- For a spicier kick, add a pinch of red pepper flakes to the marinade.
- If you don't have a spiralizer, you can use a julienne peeler to create zucchini noodles.
- You can substitute broccoli florets or asparagus for the zucchini noodles, if desired.
- Serve this dish with a side of low-carb dipping sauce, such as guacamole or hummus, for extra flavor and satisfaction.

Low-Carb Spicy Tuna Lettuce Wraps

Prep Time: 10 minutes | **Cooking Time**: 5 minutes | **Total Time**: 15 minutes | **Serving Size**: 2 lettuce wraps

Ingredients:

- 2 cans (5 oz each) tuna in water, drained and flaked
- 1/2 cup chopped celery
- 1/4 cup chopped red onion
- 1/4 cup chopped bell pepper (any color)
- 2 tablespoons mayo (use low-carb mayo if desired)
- 1 tablespoon Sriracha sauce
- 1 tablespoon lime juice
- 1/2 teaspoon chili powder
- 1/4 teaspoon salt
- 1/4 teaspoon black pepper
- 4 large romaine lettuce leaves

Optional toppings:

- Avocado slices
- Chopped cilantro
- Sesame seeds
- Lime wedges

Directions:

1. In a large bowl, combine the tuna, celery, red onion, bell pepper, mayo, Sriracha, lime juice, chili powder, salt, and pepper. Stir well to combine.
2. Wash and dry the romaine lettuce leaves.
3. Spoon the tuna mixture onto each lettuce leaf and top with your desired toppings.

Nutritional Information per serving: Calories: 350, Fat: 20g (5g saturated), Carbohydrates: 5g (3g fiber), Protein: 30g

Tips:

- For a warmer meal, pan-fry the tuna for 3-5 minutes before adding it to the bowl.
- If you're not a fan of spicy food, reduce the amount of Sriracha or omit it altogether.
- You can also use this tuna mixture to make lettuce wraps with other types of leafy greens, such as collard greens or Swiss chard.
- For a keto-friendly option, use avocado mayo instead of regular mayo.

Low-Carb Spicy Crab Cakes with Avocado Crema

Cooking Time: 10 minutes | **Prep Time**: 15 minutes | **Total Time**: 25 minutes | **Serving Size**: 4 crab cakes

Ingredients:

- 1 pound lump crab meat
- 1/2 cup almond flour
- 1/4 cup mayonnaise
- 1 tablespoon Dijon mustard
- 1/2 teaspoon Old Bay seasoning
- 1/4 teaspoon paprika
- 1/4 teaspoon cayenne pepper (optional)
- 1/4 teaspoon garlic powder
- 1/4 teaspoon onion powder
- Salt and pepper to taste
- 2 tablespoons coconut oil
- 1 avocado, halved, pitted, and mashed
- 1/4 cup lime juice
- Cilantro, chopped, for garnish
- Lime wedges, for serving

Directions:

1. Combine crabmeat, almond flour, mayonnaise, Dijon mustard, Old Bay seasoning, paprika, cayenne pepper (if using), garlic powder, onion powder, salt, and pepper in a large bowl. Gently mix until combined.
2. Divide the mixture into 4 equal portions and shape into patties. Set aside on a plate.
3. Heat coconut oil in a skillet over medium heat. Carefully place the crab cakes in the skillet and cook for 3-4 minutes per side, or until golden brown and cooked through.
4. While the crab cakes cook, prepare the avocado crema. Mash the avocado in a bowl and add lime juice. Season with salt and pepper to taste.
5. Serve crab cakes hot with avocado crema, garnished with chopped cilantro and lime wedges.

Nutritional Information per serving: Calories: 350, Fat: 25g (4g saturated), Carbohydrates: 4g (1g fiber), Protein: 30g

Tips:
- For a crispier texture, you can bread the crab cakes in crushed pork rinds before frying.
- If you don't have fresh crab meat, you can use canned crab meat, but be sure to drain it well and remove any cartilage.
- Adjust the level of spice in the crab cakes to your preference.
- This recipe is also delicious served over a bed of mixed greens or with a side of roasted vegetables.

Lobster

Cooking time: 10 minutes | **Prep time**: 10 minutes | **Total time**: 20 minutes | **Serving size**: 2

Ingredients:

- 2 frozen lobster tails, thawed
- 1 medium zucchini, spiralized
- 1 tablespoon olive oil
- 1/2 teaspoon dried oregano
- 1/4 teaspoon red pepper flakes (optional)
- Salt and black pepper to taste
- Lemon wedges, for serving

Directions:

1. Bring a pot of salted water to a boil. Add the lobster tails and cook for 5-7 minutes, or until cooked through. Remove from heat and let cool slightly.

2. Meanwhile, heat olive oil in a large skillet over medium heat. Add zucchini noodles and cook for 3-4 minutes, or until tender-crisp.

3. Stir in oregano, red pepper flakes (if using), salt, and pepper.

4. Remove lobster meat from the shells and add to the skillet with the zucchini. Toss to combine and heat through.

5. Serve immediately with lemon wedges.

Nutritional information per serving: Calories: 300, Fat: 15g, Carbs: 5g (mostly from the zucchini), Protein: 35g

Tips:

- For a richer flavor, use ghee instead of olive oil.
- Add other low-carb vegetables to the dish, such as bell peppers, mushrooms, or asparagus.
- You can also grill the lobster tails for a smoky flavor.
- Leftovers can be stored in an airtight container in the refrigerator for up to 2 days.

Baked Lemon Thyme Sardines with Zucchini Noodles

Prep Time: 15 minutes | **Cooking Time**: 20 minutes | **Total Time**: 35 minutes | **Servings**: 2

Ingredients:

- 4 sardines
- 1 tablespoon olive oil
- 1/2 lemon, sliced
- 2 fresh thyme sprigs
- Salt and pepper to taste
- 1 zucchini, spiralized into noodles
- 1/2 tablespoon chopped fresh parsley
- 1 clove garlic, minced (optional)

Directions:

1. Preheat oven to 200°C (400°F).

2. Place sardines in a baking dish. Drizzle with olive oil, top with lemon slices and thyme sprigs, and season with salt and pepper.

3. Bake for 15-20 minutes, or until sardines are cooked through and flaky.

4. While sardines are baking, spiralize the zucchini into noodles using a spiralizer or julienne peeler.

5. Heat a pan with a drizzle of olive oil (optional). Add the zucchini noodles and cook for 2-3 minutes, until slightly softened. Season with salt and pepper.

6. Serve the baked sardines on top of the zucchini noodles, sprinkle with parsley, and add minced garlic if desired.

Nutritional Information per serving: Calories: 400, Fat: 25g (good fats!), Protein: 30g, Carbs: 10g (net carbs)

Tips:

- For a smoky flavor, try grilling the sardines instead of baking.
- Add other low-carb vegetables to the zucchini noodles, such as roasted bell peppers or onions.
- Serve the sardine salad with lettuce wraps or keto bread for a more substantial meal.
- Enjoy these recipes and get creative with your own low-carb sardine dishes!

Keto-Friendly Smoked Mackerel Pate with Zucchini Noodles

Cooking Time: 10 minutes | **Prep Time**: 15 minutes | **Total Time**: 25 minutes | **Serving Size**: 2-3 people

Ingredients:

- 2 cans (5 oz each) smoked mackerel fillets in oil, drained
- 1/2 ripe avocado, mashed
- 1/4 cup lemon juice
- 1 tablespoon chopped fresh dill
- 1/2 teaspoon Dijon mustard
- Salt and pepper to taste
- 1 medium zucchini, spiralized into noodles
- Fresh dill sprigs, for garnish (optional)

Directions:

1. In a food processor or blender, combine the drained mackerel, avocado, lemon juice, dill, Dijon mustard, salt, and pepper. Blend until smooth and creamy.

2. Using a spiralizer or a julienne peeler, create zucchini noodles.

3. To assemble, divide the zucchini noodles between two plates. Top each plate with a generous dollop of the mackerel pate. Garnish with fresh dill sprigs, if desired.

Nutritional Information per serving: Calories: 350, Fat: 30g (5g saturated), Protein: 25g, Net Carbs: 5g, Fiber: 3g

Tips:

- For a spicier pate, add a pinch of cayenne pepper or red pepper flakes.
- If you don't have a food processor or blender, you can finely chop the mackerel and mash the avocado with a fork before mixing them with the other ingredients.
- Serve the pate with additional low-carb vegetables, such as cucumber slices, cherry tomatoes, or bell peppers.
- Leftover pate can be stored in an airtight container in the refrigerator for up to 3 days.

Lemon Garlic Parmesan Crusted Cod

Cooking Time: 15-20 minutes | **Prep Time**: 10 minutes | **Total Time**: 25-30 minutes | **Serving Size**: 1

Ingredients:

- 1 cod fillet (4-6 oz)
- 1/4 cup almond flour
- 1/4 cup grated Parmesan cheese
- 1 teaspoon dried parsley
- 1/2 teaspoon dried oregano
- 1/4 teaspoon garlic powder
- 1/4 teaspoon onion powder
- Salt and pepper to taste
- 1 tablespoon olive oil
- 1/2 lemon, juiced

Directions:

1. Preheat oven to 400°F (200°C). Line a baking sheet with parchment paper.
2. Pat the cod fillet dry with paper towels and season with salt and pepper.
3. In a shallow bowl, combine almond flour, Parmesan cheese, parsley, oregano, garlic powder, onion powder, salt, and pepper.
4. Drizzle the cod fillet with olive oil and sprinkle generously with the Parmesan mixture, pressing it gently into the flesh of the fish.
5. Place the cod fillet on the prepared baking sheet and drizzle with lemon juice.
6. Bake for 15-20 minutes, or until the cod is opaque and flaky.
7. Serve immediately with your favorite low-carb sides, such as roasted vegetables, steamed broccoli, or a side salad.

Nutritional Information per Serving: Calories: 400, Fat: 25 grams, Protein: 40 grams, Carbohydrates: 5 grams (2 grams net carbs)

Tips:

- For a thicker crust, you can pre-bake the cod for 5 minutes before adding the Parmesan mixture.
- You can substitute panko breadcrumbs for the almond flour, but this will increase the carbohydrate content.
- Add a pinch of cayenne pepper to the Parmesan mixture for a spicy kick.
- Leftovers can be stored in an airtight container in the refrigerator for up to 2 days.

Herb-Roasted Rainbow Trout with Lemon and Asparagus

Cooking Time: 15-20 minutes | **Prep Time**: 10 minutes | **Total Time**: 25-30 minutes | **Serving Size**: 1

Ingredients:

- 1 whole rainbow trout, cleaned and gutted
- 1 tablespoon olive oil
- 1/2 teaspoon salt
- 1/4 teaspoon black pepper
- 1 lemon, sliced
- 2 sprigs fresh rosemary
- 2 sprigs fresh thyme
- 1 bunch asparagus, trimmed

Directions:

1. Preheat oven to 425°F (220°C). Line a baking sheet with parchment paper.
2. Pat the trout dry with paper towels and brush with olive oil. Season with salt and pepper inside and out.
3. Stuff the trout cavity with lemon slices, rosemary, and thyme sprigs.
4. Place the trout on the prepared baking sheet. Arrange the asparagus around the trout. Drizzle the asparagus with a little olive oil and season with salt and pepper.
5. Roast for 15-20 minutes, or until the trout is cooked through and the asparagus is tender-crisp. The flesh should flake easily when tested with a fork.
6. Garnish with additional lemon slices and fresh herbs (optional) before serving.

Nutritional Information per serving: Calories: 350, Fat: 20g, Carbohydrates: 5g (net), Protein: 35g, Fiber: 2g

Tips:

- For extra flavor, you can marinate the trout in olive oil, lemon juice, herbs, and garlic for 30 minutes before roasting.
- If you prefer a crispier skin, broil the trout for the last 2-3 minutes of cooking time.
- Serve this dish with a side of low-carb vegetables like roasted green beans, cauliflower rice, or a simple salad.

Steamed Clams with Garlic Herb Butter

Prep time: 5 minutes | **Cooking time**: 10-12 minutes | **Total time**: 15-17 minutes | **Serving Size**: 1-2

Ingredients:

- 1 pound fresh clams, scrubbed and rinsed
- 2 tablespoons unsalted butter, melted
- 2 cloves garlic, minced
- 1/2 teaspoon dried thyme
- 1/4 teaspoon dried oregano
- 1/4 teaspoon red pepper flakes (optional)
- 1/4 cup chopped fresh parsley
- Salt and freshly ground black pepper, to taste

Directions:

1. In a large pot or Dutch oven, melt the butter over medium heat. Add the garlic, thyme, oregano, and red pepper flakes (if using). Cook for 30 seconds, until fragrant.

2. Add the clams to the pot and stir to coat in the butter mixture. Cover the pot and increase the heat to high.

3. Steam the clams for 10-12 minutes, or until they have all opened. Discard any clams that remain closed.

4. Transfer the clams to a serving platter using a slotted spoon. Pour the butter sauce over the clams and garnish with fresh parsley.

5. Season with salt and pepper to taste. Serve immediately with crusty bread or crackers (optional), if desired.

Nutritional Information per serving: Calories: 250, Fat: 18g, Carbohydrates: 2g (net), Protein: 25g

Tips:

- Be sure to use fresh clams for this recipe. Frozen clams may not open as well.
- If you don't have fresh parsley, you can substitute with chives or another fresh herb.
- For a spicier kick, add a pinch of cayenne pepper to the butter sauce.
- This recipe can be easily doubled or tripled to serve a larger crowd.

LOW-CARB BAKING

Almond Flour Bread

Prep Time: 10 minutes | **Cooking Time**: 55-70 minutes | **Total Time**: 65-80 minutes | **Serving Size**: 12 slices

Ingredients:

- 2 cups Wholesome Yum Blanched Almond Flour
- 1/4 cup Psyllium husk powder
- 1 tbsp Baking powder
- 1/2 tsp Sea salt
- 4 large Eggs (at room temperature)
- 1/4 cup Coconut oil (measured solid, then melted)
- 1/2 cup Warm water

Directions:

1. Preheat the oven to 350 degrees F (177 degrees C). Line the bottom of an 8×4 in loaf pan with parchment paper.
2. In a large bowl, use a hand mixer at high speed to beat the eggs until they double in volume.
3. In a second large bowl, mix together the almond flour, psyllium husk powder, baking powder, and sea salt
4. Beat the dry ingredients into the eggs. Beat in the melted coconut oil, then the warm water.
5. Transfer the dough to the lined baking pan. Smooth the top with a spatula.
6. Bake for 55-70 minutes, until an inserted toothpick comes out clean and the top is very hard, like a bread crust.
7. Let the bread cool in the pan for 10 minutes, then transfer it to a wire rack to cool completely.
8. Slice and enjoy!

Nutritional Information: Calories: 190 per slice, Carbohydrates: 5 grams per slice, Protein: 10 grams per slice, Fat: 13 grams per slice

Tips:

- For a sweeter bread, you can add 1 tablespoon of honey or maple syrup to the batter.
- You can also add 1/4 cup of chopped nuts or seeds to the batter.
- This bread is best stored in the refrigerator and will keep for up to 5 days.

Coconut Flour Pancakes

Prep Time: 5 minutes | **Cooking Time**: 10 minutes | **Total Time**: 15 minutes | **Serving Size**: 6 pancakes

Ingredients:

- 1/4 cup (30g) coconut flour
- 1/2 teaspoon baking powder
- 1/4 teaspoon salt
- 2 large eggs
- 2 tablespoons unsweetened almond milk
- 1 tablespoon melted coconut oil
- 1 teaspoon vanilla extract
- 1/2 teaspoon cinnamon (optional)

Directions:

1. In a medium bowl, whisk together the coconut flour, baking powder, and salt.

2. In a separate bowl, whisk together the eggs, almond milk, coconut oil, vanilla extract, and cinnamon (if using).

3. Pour the wet ingredients into the dry ingredients and stir until just combined. The batter will be thick.

4. Heat a lightly greased griddle or skillet over medium heat.

5. Pour about 1/4 cup of batter per pancake onto the griddle.

6. Cook for 3-4 minutes per side, or until golden brown.

7. Serve immediately with your favorite low-carb toppings, such as fresh berries, whipped cream, or sugar-free syrup.

Nutritional Information per pancake: Calories: 130, Fat: 8g, Carbohydrates: 4g (2g net carbs), Protein: 6g, Fiber: 2g

Tips:

- For extra fluffy pancakes, let the batter rest for 5 minutes before cooking.
- If the batter is too thick, add 1 tablespoon of almond milk at a time until it reaches the desired consistency.
- Be careful not to overcook the pancakes, as they can dry out quickly.
- These pancakes can be stored in the refrigerator for up to 3 days or frozen for up to 3 months.

Flaxseed Muffins

Cooking Time: 18-22 minutes | **Prep Time**: 10 minutes | **Total Time**: 32 minutes | **Serving Size**: 12 muffins

Ingredients:

- 1 ¼ cup ground golden flaxseed
- 1 tablespoon coconut flour
- ½ teaspoon gluten-free baking soda
- 3 tablespoons stevia sweetener (or monk fruit sweetener)
- ¾ teaspoon ground cinnamon
- ¼ teaspoon ground cloves
- ¼ teaspoon ground mace and/or nutmeg
- ¼ teaspoon pink Himalayan salt
- 4 eggs
- ⅓ cup olive oil
- ½ cup fresh or canned pumpkin puree
- ¼ cup heavy whipping cream
- 1 teaspoon vanilla extract
- 1 teaspoon lemon juice
- ¼ cup chopped pecans (optional, for topping)

Directions:

1. Preheat oven to 325°F (165°C) and line a muffin pan with 12 paper liners.
2. In a large bowl, whisk together the dry ingredients: ground flaxseed, coconut flour, baking soda, sweetener, cinnamon, cloves, mace/nutmeg, and salt.
3. In a separate bowl, whisk together the eggs, olive oil, pumpkin puree, heavy cream, vanilla extract, and lemon juice.
4. Pour the wet ingredients into the dry ingredients and stir until just combined. Do not over mix.
5. Fold in the chopped pecans (optional).
6. Divide the batter evenly among the prepared muffin cups.
7. Bake for 18-22 minutes, or until a toothpick inserted into the center comes out clean.
8. Let the muffins cool in the pan for 5 minutes, then transfer them to a wire rack to cool completely.

Nutritional Information per muffin: Calories: 180, Net Carbs: 5g, Fat: 13g, Protein: 7g, Fiber: 5g

Tips:

- For a sweeter muffin, you can add an additional tablespoon of sweetener.
- If you don't have pumpkin puree, you can substitute applesauce or mashed banana.
- You can also add other mix-ins to your muffins, such as berries, chocolate chips, or chopped nuts.
- Store leftovers in an airtight container in the refrigerator for up to 3 days.

Zucchini Bread

Prep time: 10 minutes | **Cooking time**: 50-60 minutes | **Total time**: 1 hour | **Serving size**: 12 slices

Ingredients:

- 12 ounces grated zucchini (about 1 large zucchini)
- ½ teaspoon salt
- 2 ½ cups almond flour
- ⅓ cup unflavored whey protein powder or egg white protein powder
- 2 ½ teaspoons baking powder
- 1 teaspoon cinnamon
- 3 large eggs
- ½ cup butter, melted
- ¼ – ½ cup water
- ⅓ cup dark chocolate chips, sugar-free (optional)

Directions:

1. Preheat oven to 350 degrees Fahrenheit. Grate the zucchini and place it in a colander. Sprinkle with ½ teaspoon salt and let sit for 10 minutes. Squeeze out excess moisture from the zucchini with a clean kitchen towel.
2. In a large bowl, whisk together the almond flour, protein powder, baking powder, cinnamon, and salt.
3. In a separate bowl, whisk together the eggs, melted butter, and vanilla extract.
4. Add the wet ingredients to the dry ingredients and stir until just combined. Do not over mix.
5. Stir in the drained zucchini and chocolate chips (if using).
6. Pour the batter into a greased 9x5 inch loaf pan.
7. Bake for 50-60 minutes, or until a toothpick inserted into the center comes out clean.
8. Let the bread cool in the pan for 10 minutes before slicing and serving.

Nutritional information per slice: Calories: 130, Fat: 8g, Carbs: 5g (net), Fiber: 3g, Protein: 5g

Tips:

- For a moister bread, you can add an extra ¼ cup of water to the batter.
- You can also add other mix-ins, such as chopped nuts, seeds, or shredded coconut.
- Store leftover bread in an airtight container in the refrigerator for up to 3 days.

Cheese Crackers

Prep Time: 10 minutes | **Cooking Time**: 15 minutes | **Total Time**: 25 minutes | **Serving Size**: 12 crackers

Ingredients:

- 1 cup almond flour
- 1/2 cup grated Parmesan cheese
- 1/4 cup shredded cheddar cheese
- 1/4 teaspoon salt
- 1/4 teaspoon paprika
- 1/8 teaspoon black pepper
- 2 tablespoons softened cream cheese
- 1 tablespoon cold water

Directions:

1. Preheat oven to 350°F (175°C). Line a baking sheet with parchment paper.

2. In a medium bowl, whisk together almond flour, Parmesan cheese, cheddar cheese, salt, paprika, and black pepper.

3. Add cream cheese and water, and mix until a dough forms.

4. Turn the dough out onto a lightly floured surface and roll out to about 1/4-inch thickness.

5. Cut the dough into squares or desired shapes with a pizza cutter or knife.

6. Place the crackers on the prepared baking sheet and bake for 15-20 minutes, or until golden brown.

7. Let the crackers cool on the baking sheet for a few minutes before serving.

Nutritional Information per serving: Calories: 130, Fat: 10g, Carbohydrates: 2g, Fiber: 1g, Protein: 8g

Tips:

- For a spicier cracker, add a pinch of cayenne pepper to the dough.
- You can also use other types of cheese, such as Gruyere or mozzarella.
- If the dough is too dry, add a little more water. If the dough is too sticky, add a little more almond flour.
- Store leftover crackers in an airtight container at room temperature for up to 3 days.

Avocado Brownies

Prep time: 10 minutes | **Cooking time**: 25 minutes | **Total time**: 35 minutes | **Servings**: 12 brownies

Ingredients:

- 1 ripe avocado, peeled and pitted
- 2 large eggs
- 1/2 cup almond flour
- 1/4 cup unsweetened cocoa powder
- 1/4 cup erythritol or other sugar-free sweetener
- 1/4 teaspoon baking powder
- 1/4 teaspoon salt
- 1/4 cup chopped sugar-free chocolate chips (optional)

Directions:

1. Preheat oven to 350 degrees F (175 degrees C). Line an 8x8 inch baking pan with parchment paper.

2. In a food processor or blender, combine the avocado, eggs, almond flour, cocoa powder, erythritol, baking powder, and salt. Blend until smooth.

3. Fold in the chopped chocolate chips, if using.

4. Pour the batter into the prepared baking pan and spread evenly.

5. Bake for 25-30 minutes, or until a toothpick inserted into the center comes out clean.

6. Let the brownies cool completely in the pan before cutting and serving.

Nutritional information per serving: Calories: 190, Fat: 13g, Carbohydrates: 8g (3g fiber), Protein: 4g

Tips:

- For a richer flavor, use dark chocolate chips or squares.
- You can also add other low-carb ingredients to the brownies, such as chopped nuts, seeds, or coconut flakes.
- If you don't have a food processor or blender, you can mash the avocado with a fork and then stir in the other ingredients.
- Be sure to use a sugar-free sweetener that is suitable for baking.

Flourless Peanut Butter Cookies

Prep Time: 10 minutes | **Cooking Time**: 8-10 minutes | **Total Time**: 18-20 minutes | **Serving Size**: 1 cookie

Ingredients:

- 1 cup unsweetened natural peanut butter
- 1/2 cup granulated sweetener (monk fruit, erythritol, or stevia)
- 1 large egg
- 1/4 teaspoon baking soda
- Pinch of sea salt
- Optional: 1/2 teaspoon vanilla extract

Directions:

1. Preheat oven to 350°F (175°C) and line a baking sheet with parchment paper.

2. In a large bowl, combine peanut butter, sweetener, egg, baking soda, and salt (and vanilla extract, if using). Mix until well combined and smooth.

3. Scoop out tablespoonful of dough and roll into balls. Place on the prepared baking sheet, leaving space between them.

4. Press each ball slightly with a fork to flatten, creating a crisscross pattern.

5. Bake for 8-10 minutes, or until the edges are firm and slightly golden brown.

6. Let cookies cool completely on the baking sheet before serving.

Nutritional Information per Cookie: Calories: 150, Fat: 10g, Carbohydrates: 4g (Net Carbs: 2g), Protein: 5g, Fiber: 2g

Tips:

- Use creamy peanut butter for a smoother texture. Crunchy peanut butter can be used but may result in a slightly different texture.
- Adjust the amount of sweetener to your taste preference. Keep in mind that different sweeteners have varying levels of sweetness.
- For a richer flavor, use a combination of peanut butter and almond butter.
- The cookies will be soft when they come out of the oven but will firm up as they cool.
- Store leftover cookies in an airtight container at room temperature for up to 3 days.

Low-Carb Chia Seed Pudding

Prep Time: 5 minutes | **Cooking Time**: 0 minutes | **Total Time**: 5 minutes | **Serving Size**: 1 serving

Ingredients:

- 1/4 cup chia seeds
- 1 cup unsweetened almond milk (or other low-carb milk)
- 1/2 teaspoon vanilla extract
- 1/4 teaspoon stevia powder (or other low-carb sweetener, to taste)
- Pinch of salt
- Optional toppings: fresh berries, chopped nuts, unsweetened shredded coconut, cinnamon

Directions:

1. In a bowl or jar, whisk together the chia seeds, almond milk, vanilla extract, stevia, and salt.

2. Cover the bowl or jar and refrigerate for at least 2 hours, or overnight for a thicker pudding.

3. When ready to serve, stir the pudding and top with your desired toppings.

Nutritional Information per serving: Calories: 280, Fat: 22g, Carbohydrates: 7g (3g net carbs), Fiber: 10g, Protein: 4g

Tips:

- For a richer flavor, use full-fat coconut milk instead of almond milk.
- If you don't have stevia, you can use another low-carb sweetener, such as erythritol or monk fruit sweetener.
- You can also add other flavors to your pudding, such as cocoa powder, pumpkin spice, or matcha powder.
- This pudding will keep in the refrigerator for up to 3 days.

Almond Flour Pizza Crust

Prep Time: 10 minutes | **Cooking Time**: 15-20 minutes | **Total Time**: 25-30 minutes | **Servings**: 4-6 slices

Ingredients:

- 1 1/2 cups almond flour
- 1/4 cup coconut flour
- 1/2 teaspoon baking powder
- 1/4 teaspoon salt
- 1/4 teaspoon garlic powder
- 1/4 teaspoon onion powder
- 2 large eggs
- 1 tablespoon olive oil
- Optional toppings: pizza sauce, cheese, vegetables, meat

Directions:

1. Preheat oven to 400°F (200°C). Line a baking sheet with parchment paper.
2. In a medium bowl, whisk together almond flour, coconut flour, baking powder, salt, garlic powder, and onion powder.
3. In a separate bowl, whisk together eggs and olive oil.
4. Pour the wet ingredients into the dry ingredients and mix until just combined. The dough will be sticky.
5. Transfer the dough to the prepared baking sheet and press into a 12-inch circle.
6. Bake for 15-20 minutes, or until the crust is golden brown and firm.
7. Let the crust cool slightly before topping with your favorite pizza toppings.
8. Bake for an additional 5-10 minutes, or until the cheese is melted and bubbly.
9. Slice and enjoy!

Nutritional Information per slice: Calories: 150, Fat: 10g, Carbohydrates: 4g (net carbs), Protein: 6g

Tips:

- For a crispier crust, pre-bake the crust for 10 minutes before adding toppings.
- If you don't have coconut flour, you can use all almond flour.
- You can also add other seasonings to the dough, such as Italian seasoning, red pepper flakes, or oregano.
- Get creative with your toppings! This crust is great with all sorts of different toppings.

Cauliflower Rice Pudding

Prep Time: 10 minutes | **Cooking Time**: 15 minutes | **Total Time**: 25 minutes | **Serving Size**: 4

Ingredients:

- 2 cups riced cauliflower (fresh or frozen)
- 1 cup unsweetened almond milk (or another low-carb milk)
- 1/2 cup unsweetened coconut milk (full-fat for creamier texture)
- 2 large eggs, yolks separated
- 1/4 cup sweetener (erythritol, stevia, or monk fruit sweetener)
- 1 teaspoon vanilla extract
- 1/2 teaspoon ground cinnamon
- Pinch of nutmeg (optional)
- Garnish (optional): toasted coconut flakes, chopped nuts, or berries

Directions:

1. Prepare the cauliflower: If using fresh cauliflower, cut it into florets and pulse in a food processor until they resemble rice grains. If using frozen cauliflower rice, thaw it completely and squeeze out any excess moisture with a clean kitchen towel.
2. Cook the cauliflower: In a medium saucepan, combine the riced cauliflower, almond milk, and coconut milk. Bring to a gentle simmer and cook for 5-7 minutes, or until the cauliflower is tender.
3. Whisk the egg yolks: In a separate bowl, whisk together the egg yolks and sweetener until light and fluffy.
4. Temper the eggs: Once the cauliflower is cooked, remove the pan from the heat and gradually whisk about 1/4 cup of the hot milk mixture into the egg yolks. This tempering step prevents the eggs from scrambling in the hot milk.
5. Finish the pudding: Gradually whisk the tempered egg mixture back into the saucepan with the remaining milk and cauliflower. Add the vanilla extract, cinnamon, and nutmeg (if using). Return the pan to low heat and cook, stirring constantly, for 2-3 minutes, or until the pudding thickens slightly. Do not let it boil.
6. Refrigerate and serve: Remove the pudding from the heat and let it cool slightly. Cover and refrigerate for at least 2 hours, or until chilled and set. Serve cold, garnished with your desired toppings.

Nutritional Information per Serving: Calories: 180, Fat: 13g (saturated 5g), Carbohydrates: 4g (net 2g), Fiber: 2g, Protein: 4g

Tips:

- For a richer flavor, add a tablespoon of almond butter or coconut butter to the pudding while it's simmering.
- You can adjust the sweetness to your liking. Start with less and add more to taste.
- If the pudding is too thick, add a little more milk or water. If it's too thin, simmer it for a few more minutes over low heat.
- This pudding can be stored in the refrigerator for up to 3 days.

SPECIAL OCCASION LOW-CARB RECIPES

Stuffed Portobello Mushrooms

Prep Time: 15 minutes | **Cooking Time**: 20-25 minutes | **Total Time**: 35-40 minutes | **Servings**: 4

Ingredients:

- 4 large Portobello mushrooms
- 1 tablespoon olive oil
- 1/2 teaspoon salt
- 1/4 teaspoon black pepper
- 1/2 pound ground sausage (turkey, chicken, or Italian)
- 1 small onion, diced
- 2 cloves garlic, minced
- 1/2 cup chopped spinach
- 1/4 cup shredded mozzarella cheese
- 1/4 cup chopped sun-dried tomatoes (optional)

Directions:

1. Preheat oven to 400°F (200°C).
2. Brush the Portobello mushrooms with olive oil and season with salt and pepper.
3. Carefully remove the stems and scrape out the gills with a spoon.
4. Place the mushrooms on a baking sheet and bake for 10 minutes.
5. Meanwhile, heat olive oil in a skillet over medium heat. Add the sausage and cook until browned, breaking it up with a spoon.
6. Add the onion and garlic to the skillet and cook until softened, about 5 minutes.
7. Stir in the spinach and cook until wilted.
8. Remove from heat and stir in the mozzarella cheese and sun-dried tomatoes (if using).
9. Spoon the sausage mixture into the Portobello mushrooms.
10. Bake for an additional 15-20 minutes, or until the mushrooms are tender and the cheese is melted.
11. Serve immediately.

Nutritional Information per Serving: Calories: 300, Fat: 15g, Protein: 20g, Net Carbs: 5g

Tips:

- You can also use ground beef or chicken in this recipe.
- If you don't have sun-dried tomatoes, you can use chopped fresh tomatoes or omit them altogether.
- To make this recipe vegetarian, use crumbled tofu instead of sausage.
- Serve these stuffed Portobello mushrooms with a side of low-carb salad or roasted vegetables.

Keto-Friendly Meatballs

Prep Time: 10 minutes | **Cooking Time**: 20-25 minutes | **Total Time**: 30-35 minutes | **Servings**: 12-15 meatballs

Ingredients:

- 1 pound ground beef (80/20)
- 1/2 pound ground pork
- 2 tablespoons grated Parmesan cheese
- 1/2 cup almond flour (or crushed pork rinds)
- 2 eggs
- 1 teaspoon dried oregano
- 1/2 teaspoon garlic powder
- 1/4 teaspoon onion powder
- 1/2 teaspoon salt
- 1/4 teaspoon black pepper
- 1/4 cup marinara sauce (optional)

Directions:

1. Preheat oven to 400°F (200°C). Line a baking sheet with parchment paper.

2. In a large bowl, combine ground beef, pork, Parmesan cheese, almond flour or pork rinds, eggs, oregano, garlic powder, onion powder, salt, and pepper. Mix well to combine.

3. Form the mixture into 12-15 meatballs.

4. Place the meatballs on the prepared baking sheet.

5. Bake for 20-25 minutes, or until cooked through.

6. (Optional) Brush the meatballs with marinara sauce and bake for an additional 5 minutes.

Nutritional Information per meatball: Calories: 200, Fat: 15g, Protein: 18g, Net Carbs: 2g

Tips:

- For extra flavor, add chopped fresh herbs like parsley or basil to the meatball mixture.
- You can also bake the meatballs in a single layer in an air fryer for 12-15 minutes.
- Serve the meatballs with your favorite low-carb marinara sauce, zoodles, or salad.
- Leftover meatballs can be stored in an airtight container in the refrigerator for up to 3 days.

Cauliflower Risotto

Cooking time: 20 minutes | **Prep time**: 10 minutes | **Total time**: 30 minutes | **Servings**: 4

Ingredients:

- 1 head cauliflower, cut into florets
- 1 tablespoon olive oil
- 1/2 onion, chopped
- 2 cloves garlic, minced
- 1/2 cup dry white wine (optional)
- 4 cups chicken or vegetable broth
- 1/2 cup heavy cream
- 1/2 cup grated Parmesan cheese
- Salt and pepper to taste
- Fresh herbs, such as parsley or chives, for garnish (optional)

Directions:

1. Prep the cauliflower: Pulse the cauliflower florets in a food processor until they resemble rice grains. You can also use pre-riced cauliflower if you're short on time.
2. Heat the oil: In a large skillet or Dutch oven over medium heat, heat the olive oil. Add the onion and cook until softened, about 5 minutes.
3. Add the garlic and cauliflower: Add the garlic and cook for 30 seconds until fragrant. Then, stir in the riced cauliflower and cook for 5 minutes, until slightly softened.
4. Deglaze with wine (optional): If using, pour in the white wine and scrape up any browned bits from the bottom of the pan. Let the wine simmer for 1 minute until slightly reduced.
5. Add the broth and simmer: Pour in 1 cup of the chicken or vegetable broth and bring to a simmer. Reduce heat to low and cook, stirring occasionally, until the cauliflower is tender and the broth has been absorbed, about 5-7 minutes.
6. Repeat with remaining broth: Continue adding the broth, 1/2 cup at a time, stirring constantly and letting each addition be absorbed before adding more. This slow simmering process is what helps create the creamy risotto texture.
7. Stir in cream and cheese: Once the final broth addition is absorbed, stir in the heavy cream and Parmesan cheese. Season with salt and pepper to taste.
8. Garnish and serve: Garnish with fresh herbs, if desired, and serve immediately.

Nutritional information per serving: Calories: 250, Fat: 18g, Carbohydrates: 5g (net carbs), Protein: 15g

Tips:
- For a richer flavor, use chicken broth instead of vegetable broth.
- You can add other vegetables to the risotto, such as mushrooms, peas, or spinach.
- If you don't have white wine, you can use additional broth or water.
- Leftovers can be stored in an airtight container in the refrigerator for up to 3 days.

Low-Carb Beef Wellington

Cooking Time: 45 minutes | **Prep Time**: 30 minutes | **Total Time**: 1 hour 15 minutes | **Serving**: 4-6

Ingredients:

For the Beef:
- 1 pound beef tenderloin, trimmed
- 1 tablespoon olive oil
- 1/2 teaspoon salt
- 1/4 teaspoon black pepper
- 1 tablespoon Dijon mustard

For the Mushroom Duxelle:
- 8 ounces cremini mushrooms, chopped
- 2 tablespoons butter
- 1/2 shallot, finely chopped
- 2 cloves garlic, minced
- 1/4 teaspoon dried thyme
- 1/4 cup dry white wine (optional)
- Salt and pepper to taste

For the Low-Carb Pastry:
- 8 ounces mozzarella cheese, shredded
- 3 ounces cream cheese, softened
- 1/2 cup almond flour
- 1/4 cup coconut flour
- 1 teaspoon garlic powder
- 1/2 teaspoon onion powder
- 1/2 teaspoon dried parsley
- 1/2 teaspoon baking powder
- 1/4 teaspoon baking soda
- Salt and pepper to taste
- 1 egg

Additional:
- 8 slices prosciutto
- 1 egg yolk, beaten

Directions:

1. Prepare the Beef: Preheat oven to 400°F (200°C). Heat olive oil in a large ovenproof skillet over medium-high heat. Season beef with salt and pepper. Sear on all sides for 2-3 minutes per side, until browned. Transfer to a plate and brush with Dijon mustard. Let cool slightly.

2. Make the Mushroom Duxelle: In a separate pan, melt butter over medium heat. Add shallot and garlic, cook until softened, about 5 minutes. Add mushrooms and thyme, cook until mushrooms release their liquid, about 10 minutes. If using, add white wine and cook until reduced by half. Season with salt and pepper to taste. Let cool slightly.

3. Prepare the Low-Carb Pastry: In a large bowl, combine mozzarella cheese, cream cheese, almond flour, coconut flour, garlic powder, onion powder, parsley, baking powder, baking soda, salt, and pepper. Mix until a dough forms. Add egg and knead until fully incorporated.

4. Assemble the Wellington: Lay a sheet of plastic wrap on a work surface. Spread the dough into a rectangle about 1/4-inch thick. Top with prosciutto slices, slightly overlapping. Spread the cooled mushroom Duxelle over the prosciutto. Place the cooled beef tenderloin in the center and roll up tightly, using the plastic wrap to help. Tuck in the ends of the dough to enclose the beef completely.

5. Bake and Rest: Transfer the Wellington, seam-side down, to a baking sheet lined with parchment paper. Brush with beaten egg yolk. Bake for 45 minutes, or until an internal temperature of 130°F (54°C) is reached for medium-rare. Let rest for at least 10 minutes before slicing and serving.

Nutritional Information per Serving: Calories: 420, Fat: 34g, Protein: 35g, Net Carbs: 5g

Tips:

- For a more traditional flavor, you can substitute puff pastry dough for the low-carb version. However, this will increase the carb count significantly.
- If you don't have white wine, you can use beef broth or water instead.
- To ensure even cooking, you can use a meat thermometer to check the internal temperature of the beef.
- Serve the Beef Wellington with a side of your favorite low-carb vegetables, such as roasted Brussels sprouts or asparagus.

Spaghetti Squash Carbonara

Cooking Time: 40 minutes | **Prep Time**: 15 minutes | **Total Time**: 55 minutes | **Servings**: 4

Ingredients:

- 1 medium spaghetti squash
- 4 slices bacon, chopped
- 2 cloves garlic, minced
- 2 large eggs
- 1/2 cup grated Parmesan cheese
- 1/4 cup heavy cream (optional)
- Salt and pepper to taste
- Fresh parsley, chopped (for garnish)

Directions:

1. Preheat oven to 400°F (200°C). Cut the spaghetti squash in half lengthwise and scoop out the seeds. Brush the flesh with olive oil and season with salt and pepper. Place the squash halves, cut-side down, on a baking sheet and bake for 40 minutes, or until tender.
2. While the squash is baking, cook the bacon in a large skillet over medium heat until crispy. Drain the bacon grease, leaving about 1 tablespoon in the pan. Add the garlic and cook for 30 seconds, until fragrant.
3. In a small bowl, whisk together the eggs, Parmesan cheese, and heavy cream (if using). Season with salt and pepper.
4. Once the squash is cooked, let it cool slightly. Use a fork to scrape the flesh into long strands, resembling spaghetti.
5. Add the spaghetti squash to the skillet with the bacon and garlic. Toss to combine and cook for 2 minutes over medium heat.
6. Reduce the heat to low and slowly pour in the egg mixture, whisking constantly. Continue to cook, stirring frequently, until the sauce thickens and coats the squash noodles. Do not overcook, or the eggs will become scrambled.
7. Remove from heat and stir in the cooked bacon. Garnish with fresh parsley and serve immediately.

Nutritional Information per serving: Calories: 350, Carbohydrates: 12g (net), Fat: 25g, Protein: 20g

Tips:

- For a richer flavor, use pancetta or guanciale instead of bacon.
- If you find the sauce is too thick, you can add a little bit of water or chicken broth to thin it out.
- Serve this dish with a side of roasted vegetables or a simple green salad.
- Leftovers can be stored in an airtight container in the refrigerator for up to 3 days.

Grilled Chicken Caesar Salad

Prep time: 10 minutes | **Cooking time**: 15 minutes | **Total time**: 25 minutes | **Servings**: 2

Ingredients:

For the chicken:
- 1 pound boneless, skinless chicken breasts or thighs
- 1 tablespoon olive oil
- 1/2 teaspoon salt
- 1/4 teaspoon black pepper
- 1/4 teaspoon smoked paprika (optional)

For the dressing:
- 1/4 cup mayonnaise
- 2 tablespoons lemon juice
- 1 garlic clove, minced
- 1/4 teaspoon anchovy paste (optional)
- 1/2 teaspoon Dijon mustard
- 1/4 cup grated Parmesan cheese
- Salt and black pepper to taste

For the salad:
- 4 cups romaine lettuce, chopped
- 1/2 cup cherry tomatoes, halved (optional)
- 1/4 cup sliced red onion (optional)
- 1/4 cup croutons (optional)

Directions:

1. Preheat a grill or grill pan to medium-high heat.
2. In a small bowl, whisk together the olive oil, salt, pepper, and paprika (if using). Rub the mixture onto the chicken breasts or thighs.
3. Grill the chicken for 5-7 minutes per side, or until cooked through.
4. While the chicken is cooking, whisk together the mayonnaise, lemon juice, garlic, anchovy paste (if using), Dijon mustard, and Parmesan cheese in a small bowl. Season with salt and pepper to taste.
5. To assemble the salad, divide the romaine lettuce between two plates. Top with the grilled chicken, cherry tomatoes (if using), red onion (if using), and croutons (if using). Drizzle with the Caesar dressing and serve immediately.

Nutritional information per serving: Calories: 450, Fat: 30g, Carbohydrates: 5g (net), Protein: 40g

Tips:
- You can also use pre-cooked chicken for this recipe. Simply shred or slice the chicken and add it to the salad.
- If you don't have anchovy paste, you can use Worcestershire sauce instead.
- To make the salad even more filling, you can add some avocado or chopped nuts.
- For a truly low-carb version, omit the croutons.

I hope you enjoy this recipe!

Keto-Friendly Crab Cakes

Cooking Time: 8-10 minutes | **Prep Time**: 15 minutes | **Total Time**: 25-30 minutes | **Servings**: 6 crab cakes

Ingredients:

- 8 ounces lump crab meat, drained and picked over
- 1 large egg, beaten
- 2 tablespoons mayonnaise
- 1 tablespoon Dijon mustard
- 1 tablespoon lemon juice
- 1/2 teaspoon Old Bay seasoning
- 1/4 teaspoon salt
- 1/4 teaspoon black pepper
- 1/4 cup almond flour, blanched and finely ground
- 1 tablespoon chopped fresh parsley
- 2 tablespoons avocado oil or ghee

Directions:

1. In a large bowl, gently combine the crab meat, egg, mayonnaise, Dijon mustard, lemon juice, Old Bay seasoning, salt, pepper, almond flour, and parsley. Mix just until incorporated, being careful not to over mix or break up the crab meat.
2. Heat the avocado oil or ghee in a large skillet over medium heat. Using a spoon or ice cream scoop, form the crab mixture into 6 equal patties.
3. Gently place the crab cakes in the hot oil and cook for 4-5 minutes per side, or until golden brown and crispy. Alternatively, you can bake the crab cakes on a preheated baking sheet at 400°F for 15-20 minutes, flipping halfway through.
4. Serve immediately with your favorite low-carb dipping sauce, such as remoulade, tartar sauce, or a simple lemon wedge. Enjoy!

Nutritional Information per Serving: Calories: 240, Fat: 18g, Protein: 20g, Net Carbs: 2g

Tips:

- For a richer flavor, add a tablespoon of minced shallots or chives to the mixture.
- If the crab mixture seems too wet, add another tablespoon of almond flour.
- Don't overcook the crab cakes, or they will become dry and tough.
- Leftovers can be stored in an airtight container in the refrigerator for up to 2 days. Reheat gently in a skillet or oven.

Cabbage Wrapped Tacos

Cook Time: 20 minutes | **Prep Time**: 15 minutes | **Total Time**: 35 minutes | **Serving Size**: 4 tacos

Ingredients:

- 1 head of Napa cabbage
- 1 pound ground beef (90% lean or higher)
- 1/2 onion, diced
- 1 bell pepper (any color), diced
- 2 cloves garlic, minced
- 1 teaspoon chili powder
- 1/2 teaspoon cumin
- 1/4 teaspoon smoked paprika
- Salt and pepper to taste
- 1/2 avocado, mashed
- 1 tablespoon lime juice
- Cilantro, chopped (optional)
- Hot sauce (optional)

Directions:

1. Prep the cabbage: Carefully remove the outer leaves of the cabbage head. Slice off the bottom thick part of the stem to create a flat base. Gently peel off 8 large leaves, keeping them whole. Set aside.
2. Cook the ground beef: In a large skillet over medium heat, brown the ground beef with the onion and bell pepper until cooked through. Drain any excess fat.
3. Season the filling: Add the garlic, chili powder, cumin, paprika, salt, and pepper to the cooked beef mixture. Stir well to combine and cook for an additional minute.
4. Warm the cabbage leaves: Fill a large pot with water and bring to a simmer. Carefully dunk each cabbage leaf in the hot water for 30 seconds to soften them. Remove with tongs and transfer to a plate lined with paper towels to drain.
5. Make the avocado sauce: Mash the avocado with the lime juice. Season with salt and pepper to taste.
6. Assemble the tacos: Place a spoonful of cooked beef mixture on each cabbage leaf. Top with avocado sauce, chopped cilantro (optional), and a drizzle of hot sauce (optional). Fold the sides of the leaf over the filling to create a wrap.
7. Serve immediately and enjoy!

Nutritional Information per serving: Calories: 350, Fat: 20g (3g saturated), Carbohydrates: 10g (5g fiber), Protein: 30g

Tips:

- You can substitute ground turkey or chicken for the ground beef.
- Feel free to add other vegetables to the filling, such as shredded carrots, zucchini, or mushrooms.
- Add a dollop of Greek yogurt or sour cream for an extra creamy touch.
- For a spicier kick, add a diced jalapeño pepper to the filling.
- These cabbage wraps are best enjoyed fresh but can be stored in the refrigerator for up to 24 hours.

Low-Carb Cheesecake

Prep Time: 15 minutes | **Cooking Time**: 50-55 minutes | **Total Time**: 1 hour 10 minutes | **Servings**: 10-12 slices

Ingredients:

Crust:
- 1 1/2 cups almond flour
- 1/4 cup powdered sweetener (erythritol or monk fruit)
- 1/4 cup melted butter
- 1/4 teaspoon vanilla extract

Filling:
- 24 ounces full-fat cream cheese, softened
- 1 cup sour cream
- 3 large eggs
- 3/4 cup powdered sweetener
- 1 tablespoon lemon juice
- 1 teaspoon vanilla extract

Optional toppings:
- Whipped cream, berries, sugar-free chocolate sauce

Directions:

1. Preheat oven to 350°F (175°C). Line the bottom of a 9-inch spring form pan with parchment paper.
2. Prepare the crust: In a medium bowl, combine almond flour, sweetener, melted butter, and vanilla extract. Mix until crumbly. Press the mixture evenly into the bottom of the prepared pan. Bake for 10 minutes, then let cool slightly.
3. Make the filling: In a large bowl, beat the cream cheese and sour cream until smooth. Add the eggs, sweetener, lemon juice, and vanilla extract. Beat until just combined, being careful not to over mix.
4. Pour the filling over the cooled crust. Tap the pan gently on the counter to release any air bubbles.
5. Bake for 50-55 minutes, or until the cheesecake is almost set but still slightly jiggly in the center. Turn off the oven and leave the cheesecake inside with the door slightly ajar for 30 minutes.
6. Refrigerate for at least 4 hours, or overnight, before serving.

Nutritional Information per slice: Calories: 280, Fat: 23g (16g saturated), Protein: 8g, Carbohydrates: 3g (2g net carbs), Fiber: 1g, Sugar: 0g

Tips:
- For a richer flavor, use full-fat cream cheese and sour cream.
- Let the cheesecake cool completely before slicing to prevent cracking.
- If you don't have a spring form pan, you can use a regular pie pan, but the crust will be slightly thicker.
- Get creative with toppings! Sugar-free chocolate sauce, berries, or a sprinkle of chopped nuts are all delicious options.

Keto-Friendly Chocolate Mousse

Prep time: 10 minutes | **Cooking time**: 0 minutes | **Total time**: 10 minutes | **Servings**: 4

Ingredients:

- 1 cup heavy cream
- 1/2 cup unsweetened cocoa powder
- 1/4 cup erythritol sweetener (or sweetener of your choice)
- 1/2 teaspoon vanilla extract
- Pinch of salt

Directions:

1. In a large bowl, whip the heavy cream until stiff peaks form.

2. In a separate bowl, whisk together the cocoa powder, erythritol sweetener, vanilla extract, and salt.

3. Gently fold the dry ingredients into the whipped cream until just combined. Be careful not to over mix, as this can make the mousse tough.

4. Divide the mousse among four serving dishes and chill for at least 2 hours before serving.

Nutritional information per serving: Calories: 280, Fat: 28g, Carbohydrates: 2g (net), Protein: 2g

Tips:

- For an extra rich flavor, use melted dark chocolate instead of cocoa powder.
- You can also add a pinch of espresso powder or instant coffee to the dry ingredients for a mocha flavor.
- Top your mousse with a dollop of whipped cream, grated chocolate, or a few raspberries for an extra decadent treat.

WEEK 1

Day 1:
Breakfast: Avocado and Bacon Egg Cups
Lunch: Grilled Chicken Salad
Snack: Zucchini Fries

Day 2:
Breakfast: Spinach and Feta Omelette
Lunch: Zucchini Noodles with Pesto
Snack: Cucumber Bites

Day 3:
Breakfast: Keto Pancakes
Lunch: Cauliflower Fried Rice
Snack: Deviled Eggs

Day 4:
Breakfast: Chia Seed Pudding
Lunch: Turkey Lettuce Wraps
Snack: Baked Buffalo Cauliflower Bites

Day 5:
Breakfast: Baked Egg Muffins
Lunch: Eggplant Parmesan
Snack: Cheese Crisps

Day 6:
Breakfast: Greek Yogurt Parfait
Lunch: Cabbage and Beef Stir-Fry
Snack: Stuffed Mushrooms

Day 7:
Breakfast: Low-Carb Smoothie
Lunch: Cauliflower Crust Pizza
Snack: Guacamole with Veggie Sticks

WEEK 2

Day 8:
Breakfast: Smoked Salmon Roll-Ups
Lunch: Shrimp Avocado Salad
Snack: Crispy Bacon-Wrapped Asparagus

Day 9:
Breakfast: Cauliflower Hash Browns
Lunch: Greek Salad with Grilled Chicken
Snack: Antipasto Skewers

Day 10:
Breakfast: Keto Breakfast Burrito
Lunch: Grilled Chicken Salad
Snack: Cauliflower Hummus with Veggie Dippers

Day 11:
Breakfast: Coconut Flour Waffles
Lunch: Zucchini Noodles with Pesto
Snack: Zucchini Fries

Day 12:
Breakfast: Caprese Salad
Lunch: Turkey Lettuce Wraps
Snack: Cucumber Bites

Day 13:
Breakfast: Keto Breakfast Casserole
Lunch: Eggplant Parmesan
Snack: Deviled Eggs

Day 14:
Breakfast: Egg and Bacon Roll-Ups
Lunch: Cauliflower Crust Pizza
Snack: Cheese Crisps

GROCERY SHOPPING LIST ON LOW-CARB DIET

Proteins:
Chicken breasts
Ground turkey or chicken
Salmon fillets
Shrimp
Eggs
Bacon
Ground beef
Deli turkey or chicken slices

Vegetables:
Spinach
Avocados
Zucchini
Cauliflower
Broccoli
Cucumber
Bell peppers
Eggplant
Cherry tomatoes
Asparagus
Mushrooms
Lettuce (for salads and lettuce wraps)
Fresh herbs (such as basil, cilantro, parsley)

Fruits:
Berries (e.g., strawberries, blueberries, raspberries) - in moderation

Dairy and Alternatives:
Greek yogurt (unsweetened)
Cheese (cheddar, mozzarella, feta, etc.)
Unsweetened almond milk or coconut milk
Cream cheese
Butter
Heavy cream

Nuts and Seeds:
Almonds
Walnuts
Pecans
Chia seeds
Flaxseeds

Flours and Baking Ingredients:
Almond flour
Coconut flour
Baking powder
Vanilla extract
Sugar substitutes (stevia, erythritol, and monk fruit)

Pantry Staples:
Olive oil
Coconut oil
Avocado oil
Vinegar (apple cider vinegar, balsamic vinegar)

Soy sauce or tamari (for gluten-free option)
Spices and herbs (such as garlic powder, onion powder, paprika, cumin, oregano, basil)

Condiments and Sauces:
Sugar-free tomato sauce or marinara sauce
Mustard
Hot sauce
Low-carb salad dressings (check labels for added sugars)

Frozen Foods:
Frozen berries
Frozen cauliflower rice
Frozen spinach
Frozen broccoli

Miscellaneous:
Low-carb tortillas or wraps (if desired)
Coconut flakes (unsweetened)
Dark chocolate (85% or higher cocoa content, in moderation)

Remember to check labels for added sugars and hidden carbohydrates, especially in packaged and processed foods. Buying fresh and whole foods is generally the best approach for a low-carb diet. Adjust quantities based on your meal plan and personal preferences.

FREQUENTLY ASKED QUESTIONS

What is a low-carb diet? A low-carb diet is a dietary plan that limits the consumption of carbohydrates, often to encourage weight reduction, regulate blood sugar levels, or enhance overall health. Carbohydrates are reduced while protein and fat consumption are prioritized.

What foods are permitted on a low-carb diet? Foods permitted on a low-carb diet often include non-starchy vegetables, meat, poultry, fish, eggs, nuts, seeds, healthy fats like olive oil and avocado, and some dairy products like cheese and Greek yogurt. Foods heavy in carbs including bread, pasta, rice, and sweet snacks are restricted or avoided.

Are all carbs unhealthy on a low-carb diet? Not all carbs are considered detrimental on a low-carb diet. While refined carbs like white bread and sugary meals are banned, non-starchy vegetables, berries, and other high-fiber foods are recommended because of their decreased influence on blood sugar levels.

How many carbohydrates should I consume on a low-carb diet? The quantity of carbohydrates permitted on a low-carb diet might vary based on individual characteristics such as age, gender, exercise level, and weight reduction objectives. However, normal ranges for daily carbohydrate consumption on a low-carb diet may range from 20 to 100 grams per day.

What are the possible advantages of a low-carb diet? Some possible advantages of a low-carb diet include weight reduction, better blood sugar management, lower risk of type 2 diabetes, improved cholesterol levels, and greater sensations of fullness and satisfaction.

Are there any hazards or negative effects linked with a low-carb diet? Some individuals may have early negative effects after beginning a low-carb diet, such as tiredness, headache, dizziness, or constipation. Long-term adherence to extremely low-carb diets may also raise concerns about nutritional deficits if not adequately balanced.

Can I still work out on a low-carb diet? Yes, you can still work out on a low-carb diet. While some people may suffer a brief decline in performance during the early transition period, many individuals find that their energy levels normalize with time. Consuming appropriate protein and healthy fats may assist promote physical activity and recuperation.

Is a low-carb diet appropriate for everyone? A low-carb diet may not be suited for everyone, particularly those with specific medical issues or dietary limitations. It's vital to check with a healthcare physician or trained dietitian before beginning any new diet plan, particularly if you have underlying health issues or are pregnant or nursing.

GLOSSARY

1. **Carbohydrates (Carbs):** Macronutrients found in foods including grains, fruits, vegetables, and dairy products. They are the body's major source of energy. On a low-carb diet, carbohydrate consumption is reduced to varied degrees.

2. **Ketosis:** A metabolic state in which the body transitions from utilizing carbs as its major fuel source to using fat and ketones for energy. Ketosis is commonly attained on extremely low-carb diets, such as the Ketogenic diet.

3. **Ketogenic Diet (Keto Diet):** An extremely low-carb, high-fat diet meant to induce ketosis. It generally entails ingesting fewer than 50 grams of carbs per day to boost fat burning and weight reduction.

4. **Net Carbs:** The total carbs in a meal minus the fiber and some sugar alcohols that are not completely absorbed by the body. Some low-carb diets count net carbohydrates instead of total carbs when measuring carbohydrate consumption.

5. **Dietary Fiber:** The indigestible portion of plant foods that helps improve digestive health, control blood sugar levels and assist weight management. Foods rich in fiber are generally promoted on low-carb diets.

6. **Glycemic Index (GI):** A measure of how rapidly carbs in a diet boost blood sugar levels. Foods with a low glycemic index are digested and absorbed more slowly, leading to more stable blood sugar levels.

7. **Insulin:** A hormone generated by the pancreas that helps control blood sugar levels by promoting the absorption of glucose into cells for energy. Low-carb diets may help increase insulin sensitivity and lower insulin levels in certain people.

8. **Macronutrients (Macros):** The three basic nutrients that supply energy to the body: carbs, proteins, and fats. Low-carb diets often include altering the ratio of macronutrients to encourage fat reduction or other health advantages.

9. **Glucose:** A simple sugar that serves as the principal source of energy for the body's cells. It is produced from the breakdown of carbs in the diet and is controlled by insulin.

10. **Sugar Alcohols:** Sweeteners often used in sugar-free and low-carb goods as substitutes for sugar. Examples include erythritol, xylitol, and sorbitol. They contain fewer calories and a lower influence on blood sugar levels than ordinary sugar.

11. **Lipogenesis:** The process by which the body turns extra dietary carbs into fat for storage. Restricting carbohydrate intake on a low-carb diet may assist minimize Lipogenesis and boost fat burning.

12. **Glucagon:** A hormone generated by the pancreas that helps control blood sugar levels by increasing the release of glucose from the liver when blood sugar levels are low. It has the opposite action of insulin.